Once
a
Runner

A Novel

John L. Parker, Jr.

Scribner

New York   London   Toronto   Sydney

SCRIBNER
A Division of Simon & Schuster, Inc.
1230 Avenue of the Americas
New York, NY 10020

First Scribner trade paperback edition April 2010

SCRIBNER and design are registered trademarks of
The Gale Group, Inc., used under license
by Simon & Schuster, Inc., the publisher of this work.

For information about special discounts for bulk purchases,
please contact Simon & Schuster Special Sales at
1-866-506-1949 or business@simonandschuster.com

The Simon & Schuster Speakers Bureau can bring authors to your
live event. For more information or to book an event contact
the Simon & Schuster Speakers Bureau at 1-866-248-3049
or visit our website at www.simonspeakers.com.

Designed by Suet Y. Chong
Text set in Baskerville 2

Manufactured in the United States of America

21 23 25 27 29 30 28 26 24 22

Library of Congress Control Number: 2008024255

ISBN 978-1-4165-9788-9
ISBN 978-1-4165-9789-6 (pbk)
ISBN 978-1-4165-9791-9 (ebook)

Also by John L. Parker, Jr.

Again to Carthage

Runners & Other Dreamers

Marty Liquori's Guide for the Elite Runner
(with Marty Liquori)

Run Down Fired Up and Teed Off

And Then the Vulture Eats You
(editor)

Heart Monitor Training for the Compleat Idiot

Praise for *Once a Runner*

"By far the most accurate fictional portrayal of the world of the serious runner . . . a marvelous description of the way it really is."
—*Sports Illustrated*

"Time has not taken a toll on this gem. . . . Runners will find inspirational passages everywhere that they will want to save."
—*Star Tribune*

"Don't let twenty years of pent-up anticipation and expectation ruin your run through this book. It's paced a little like a marathon—controlled start, strong finish. . . . Don't think you have to be a world-class athlete to connect with Quenton Cassidy and love this book. If you've ever trained and competed at your own highest level, you'll get this guy."
—*The Kansas City Star*

"A finely crafted work of fiction."
—*St. Petersburg Times*

"Part training manual, part religious tract, part love story, and all about running, *Once a Runner* is so inspiring it could be banned as a performance-enhancing drug."
—Benjamin Cheever, author of *Strides: Running Through History with an Unlikely Athlete,* in *Runner's World*

"*Once a Runner*'s famed ability to convey the thrill of the sport leaves its mark."
—*St. Louis Post-Dispatch*

"Inspirational."
—*Chicago Sun-Times*

This book is for Jack Bacheler and Frank Shorter,
old friends, great runners. In fond remembrance, fellows,
of many Trials and many Miles . . .

How did I know you ran the mile in 4:30 in high school? That's easy. *Everyone* ran the mile in 4:30 in high school.

—Frank Shorter, *out running somewhere*, circa 1969

Once . . .

THE NIGHT JOGGERS were out as usual.

The young man could see dim figures on the track even in this pale light, slowly pounding round and round the most infinite of footpaths. There would be, he knew, plump, determined-looking women slogging along while fleshy knees quivered. They would occasionally brush damp hair fiercely from their eyes and dream of certain cruel and smiling emcees: bikinis, ribbon-cuttings, and the like. And then, of course, tennis with white-toothed males, wild tangos in the moonlight.

And men too of various ages and levels of dilapidation, perhaps also grinding out secret fantasies (did they picture themselves a Peter Snell held back only by fat or fear as they turned their ninety-second quarters?).

The young man stood outside the fence for a few moments

while moths attacked the streetlight dustily, leaving him in a dim spotlight of swirling shadows. He loved early fall in Florida's Panhandle. Leaves would be turning elsewhere but here the hot breath of summer held forth. In the moist warmth there was a slight edge, though, a faint promise of cooler air hanging in the treetops and close to the Spanish moss. He picked up his small travel bag and went in the gate, walking clockwise on the track toward the white starting post at the head of the first turn. The joggers ignored the stranger in street clothes and he likewise paid them no attention. They would always be there.

The high-jump pit had been rearranged, a new section of bleachers added, a water jump installed for the steeplechase. But mostly it looked the same as it did four years ago, the same as a four-hundred-and-forty-yard oval probably will always look to one who knows a quarter of a mile by the inches.

The Games were over for this time around. He knew quite well that for him they were over for good. Four years is a very long time in some circles; in actual time—real-world time, as that of shopkeepers, insurance sellers, compounders of interest, and so on—it is perhaps not long at all. But in his own mind Time reposed in peculiar receptacles; to him the passing of one minute took on all manner of rare meaning. A minute was one fourth of a four-minute mile, a coffee spoon of his days and ways.

As with many of the others, he had no idea what he would be doing now that it was all over. It was such a demanding thing, so final, so cathartic, that most of them simply never thought beyond it. They were scattered around the world now, he supposed, doing pretty much what he was doing at this moment: thinking everything over, tallying gains and losses.

He was going to have to pick up the thread of a normal life again and although he did not exactly know why, he had to start by coming back here, back to the greenhouse warmth of the Panhandle, back to this very quarter-mile oval that still held his long-dried sweat. Back to September, the month of promises.

He put his bag down by the pole-vault pit, looked uptrack to make sure no one was coming, and then walked up to the starting line. God, he thought, one more time on the line.

In lane one he stood very still, looking down at his street shoes (joggers now going around him with curious glances) and tried to conjure up the feeling. After a moment a trace of it came to him and he knew that was all there would be. You can remember it, he told himself, but you cannot experience it again like this. You have to be satisfied with the shadows. Then he thought about how it was in the second and third laps and decided that the shadows were sometimes quite enough.

He was twenty-six years, five months, and two days old, and though as he stood there on the starting line he felt quite a bit older than that, the muscles that rippled up and down inside his trouser leg could have only been the result, biologically speaking, of more thousands of miles than he cared to think about all at one time.

He tried to focus blurred emotions, a metaphysical photographer zeroing in on hard edges to align in the center square. What was this he was feeling now, nostalgia? Regret? His mind double-clutched, asked the musical question: Am . . . I . . . buh-loooo?

He could not tell. He realized again how adept he had become at not being able to tell such things. His emotions had calluses like feet.

The starter would tell them to stand tall, so he stood tall for a moment there in the night. There would be the set command and then the gun. He took a deep breath and began walking into the turn in the familiar counterclockwise direction, the way of all races, and thought: the first lap is lost in a flash of adrenaline and pounding hooves . . .

2.

Doobey Hall

D OOBEY HALL was one of those ancient resonant wooden buildings that seemed to hold the oils and essences of those who had lived there over the years. Like an old cloth easy chair, it was musty but comfortable.

As with many structures that had at one time been someone's home, it managed to retain a certain familial warmth amid the current institutional clamor. It thumped and boomed hollowly rather than clicking in the bony staccato manner of more modern, more efficient dwellings.

Having once housed Kernsville mayor Hiram "Sidecar" Doobey and his various clamoring kindred, the large friendly house had been used during recent years to shelter thirty-some members of Southeastern University's grateful track team. Located a merciful two blocks from the campus proper, the edifice

emitted from morning to night a steady but unpredictable caco-
phony of barely human yelps, primordial shrieks, and off-key
fragments of current hit songs, all courtesy of a singular group of
young sapiens whose main function in life was to run, jump, and
toss heavy objects about. And to do so far better than, well, ordinary mortals. The net available energy required to produce a
seventy-foot shot put or a seven-foot high jump just occasionally
would not be contained by mere wood and plaster.

Walls trembled and there were eerie goings-on.

OLD SIDECAR DOOBEY—deceased for years now—would have
been tickled pink. His nickname was an artifact of those carefree
Depression days of yesteryear when on a Saturday night for pure
diversion Doobey would down about three quarters of a jar of the
local untaxed beverage, scoop up his tiny startled wife—a pretty,
round-eyed thing named Emma Lee—deposit her in the sidecar
of his 1932 Harley Davidson seventy-four-inch flathead, and proceed to more or less terrorize nearby herds of grazing cattle.

"Woman," he would tell her, "we fixin' to do some *night rid-
in'*!" His wild green eyes held her for a moment like a light.

"Eeeeee!" she said.

This is not to imply that Sidecar was an outlaw exactly, since
he owned most of the cows in Kalhoun County (and a good deal
of the land and several sensitive mortgages for that matter). He
was just what some folks called "lively." Sidecar was one of those
raw, energetic men who understand very early in life which
levers and pulleys really worked and which were just for show.
And he also understood that the whole shebang was most certainly going to come to a grinding halt one fine day. Irretrievably,
he suspected.

The only time he found himself in any kind of trouble worthy
of the name was one night when he got particularly rowdy, broke
down some fences, and (Emma Lee squeaking like a wounded

bat) went roaring into downtown Kernsville to "strafe the goll-danged pigeons" while sad-eyed old codgers sat around the courthouse square watching in wrinkled amusement.

"Lawd, Sheriff, I su*wa*nee . . . I *lawd* don't know why I get so mean sometimes," he said with true regret the morning after his actual arrest. He held his shaggy, throbbing head in his hands.

"Well, Daddy," said the sheriff, "people is beginning to talk, and that's a fack." Sheriff William "Boots" Doobey was his eldest.

"What I cain't quite figure out," continued the lawman, "is why you always want to go and take Mama with you."

Sidecar perked up suddenly. "Why," he cackled savagely, "she enjoys the *pure T hell out of it*!"

It was perhaps reflective of the university town's collective sense of humor when it elected Sidecar mayor a year later. He had run on a platform of throw the bastards out, interesting only because the bastards were, nearly without exception, his own blood kin. True to form, he threw the bastards out.

Sidecar's election had been like much of his life, a prize thrust upon him almost without the asking. The old man's one deep hurt came when his youngest boy, born when Sidecar was fifty-two and Emma Lee nearly forty, turned out to be something of an ordinary klutz. Boots could have had a West Point appointment, Sheryl Ann was a Georgia Tech homecoming queen (before dropping out to marry a middle linebacker). It touched a deep, painful place in his breast when Sidecar anxiously watched the youngster, more like a grandson really, trying to master the elementary gearshift configuration of the big John Deere tractor. When the child was stymied by a cousin half his age at a simple card game, Sidecar wandered out into his fields and wept with rage.

At that moment Sidecar decided, being a man of large concepts as well as a patron of irony, to get for this slightly addled child that which his other children lacked (and didn't want for that matter): academic status. Years later, this curious task would be accomplished in the way that difficult or impossible objectives are generally accomplished by men of great power and lesser scruples, which is to say on the sly. He deeded over to Southeastern University (which desperately needed space for a nascent entomology department) the house he had occupied for seven years as mayor. The deed contained the usual boiler-plate: "In exchange for ten dollars and other good and lawful consideration . . ." The nature of the other good and lawful con-sideration was known only to Sidecar himself, his lawyer, and the president-designate of the school, the Honorable Steven C. Prigman, late of Florida's august supreme court. At that time Emma Lee was five years in her grave and old Sidecar wanted to get away from "downgoddamntown politics" and back to his ranch where he could "at least goddamn well die with the hon-est smell of fresh dung and hay in my nostrils." He didn't men-tion that he was actually toying with the notion of reviving the ancient and beloved Harley, then rusting under a paint-spattered canvas tarp in the barn.

His youngest would have to go through the motions of attend-ing the university, so the formal conferring of the degree would not take place for another four years. Sidecar mucked around the ranch, got in his foreman's hair, bought a fifty-five-acre pecan grove, and was finally persuaded to purchase a package tour deal to several Mexican cities of interest. He returned raving about the regenerative properties of certain cactus distillates and hint-ing darkly about the "im-and-ex port bidness."

On the scholastic scene things went without a hitch and the old man lived to see his boy, dazed and sweating like a field hand in his cap and gown, marching numbly to "Pomp and Circum-stance." Entomology outgrew Doobey Hall in a few years and the track team, delighted to a man, inherited it. Sidecar passed on soon thereafter but it was said he tried to kick his way out of the coffin on the way to Jesus Walks Among Us Acres.

A good bit of Doobey folklore was known in and around Kernsville and accounted for no small amount of graffiti scattered about the campus. Bold red letters on the side of the old field house one semester warned ominously: SIDECAR LIVES!

Hiram Sidecar Doobey, lusty gallivanter, bovine terrorist, and ball twister par excellence, ended up as kind of a regional backwoods Kilroy.

And the last male heir of his body, he of the dim wit, bogus degree, and unaccountable penchant for hurting insects, his youngest son, Dick Doobey, ended up as the head football coach.

3

The Morning Run

ON THE THIRD FLOOR of Doobey Hall was the room in which Dick Doobey had slept as a child. Now its battered oak door held two three-by-five index cards neatly thumbtacked one atop the other.

The top one said in Smith Corona pica:

```
If you can fill the unforgiving minute
With sixty seconds' worth of distance run—
Yours is the Earth and everything that's in it,
And—which is more—you'll be a Man, my son!
—Rudyard Kipling, 1892
```

The other card read:

Rudyard Kipling was a 4:30 miler.

—Quenton Cassidy, 1969

Inside the room, the one true Quenton Cassidy slept fitfully as dawn approached. In a damp orb of his own worst fears, he nightmared with a certain grace. It was an old and familiar theme with him: the last lap of a footrace found him being soundly thrashed by every man on the track. He was running in peanut butter up to his waist as they all glided by easily. He tried to use his hands to grab something to propel himself along, but it was useless. What was wrong here? Was his training inadequate? Where was his kick?

Mercifully, he awoke. Before the alarm, moist from his fretting, but forgetting the dream quickly. He sat on the edge of the bed wiggling his toes thoughtfully as the cobwebs of anxiety slowly melted away in his shaggy head. In the waking world his whole being centered around covering ground quickly on foot. At this he really had no equals save a few dozen others scattered about the country and world who also woke to such disquieting dreams. Quenton Cassidy knew every one of them by name.

Wearing only the weightless nylon shorts he slept in, he ambled stiffly to the dawn-lit window and stood momentarily, drowsily enjoying the pale orange-yellow glow that suffused the blackjack oaks outside his room. A slight breeze was chilly enough to raise goose bumps on sleep-warm flesh. He did not much like this early morning business, but the idea of forgoing it, even for one morning, never crossed his mind.

Quenton Cassidy was six foot two, his meager 167 pounds stretched across his frame in the manner dictated by the searing daily necessities of his special task. Beneath the tight skin, a smooth musculature glided with fluid ease, giving the impression of elastic, lightweight power: a featherless view of a young falcon.

There were no inefficient corners or bulges; the form was

sharply chiseled as if from sand-worn driftwood, fluted with oblique angles and long, tapering ridges, thin products of his care. Even now, as he stood perfectly still in the early morning glow, inverted-teardrop thighs and high bunched calves suggested only motion: smooth effortless speed.

Stretching with a lovely kind of pain, he turned from the window and sat again on the edge of the rumpled bed to put on his worn Adidas Gazelle training shoes. His face was ruddy, even in the soft light, with a Scandinavian nose and sharp cheekbones; its attractiveness was debatable. Ragged brownish hair, bleached by hours of sun, tumbled in no particular pattern as he double-knotted his shoes. He washed his hands in the sink (the shoelaces, repositories of ancient sweat, smelled like something that had died behind the refrigerator) and with a grunt he was out the door and gone.

Quenton Cassidy was a miler.

OUT IN THE EARLY MORNING STREETS, the small group of runners made its way down University Avenue and turned north on Thirty-fourth Street; they would traverse a large seven-mile square known interchangeably as "the Morning Loop," "the Seven-Mile Course," or "the Bacon Strip" (for a series of undulating hills). Cassidy ran in the back of the pack with a loose stride that approached awkwardness. For a miler the 6:30 pace was a stumble, but with his accumulated fatigue he wanted nothing more challenging. He chatted quietly with Jerry Mizner, a thinner and darker runner who had the look of a true distance man. He and Cassidy had been through what they now called the "Trial of Miles." As with shipwreck survivors, hostages, and others in dire circumstances, duress fosters an unsentimental kind of intimacy. At times Cassidy and Mizner seemed to be able to read each other's minds.

"I don't think it can be done, really," Mizner said.

"It's absolutely true. I can sleep for at least the first half mile. I'm sure of it. They say soldiers can march when—"

"Nah . . ."

"Well, it *feels* like I'm sleeping, that's good enough for me."

"Feeling and doing are different. Plato said that. Or Hugh Hefner. One of the philosophers anyway."

For Cassidy there was no joy at all in this morning routine. He slept hard and woke slowly. The morning people who claimed to like these dawn-lit forays really annoyed him. But the gentle conversation made it easier, a social occasion of sorts, for just as rank has its privileges so indeed does the barely comprehensible conditioning of good distance runners. They gab like magpies.

At paces that might stun and dismay the religious jogger, the runners easily kept up all manner of chatter and horseplay. When they occasionally blew by a huffing fatty or an aging road runner, they automatically toned down the banter to avoid overwhelming, to preclude the appearance of showboating (not that they slowed in the slightest). They in fact respected these distant cousins of the spirit, who, among all people, had some modicum of insight into their own milieu. But the runners resembled them only in the sense that a puma resembles a pussycat. It is the difference between stretching lazily on the carpet and prowling the jungle for fresh red meat.

"I suppose we'll soon know who's nice and rested from the weekend," Cassidy said. They were nearing the halfway point.

"Three guesses," said Mizner.

Despite the standing prohibition against racing during long runs, a practice that rapidly got out of hand, a younger runner would occasionally light out for cheap glory.

"Get a load," Cassidy said, gesturing ahead. Mizner looked up and gave Cassidy a grin and an I'll-be-fugged shrug.

"Monday Morning Scalders," Mizner said jauntily. The reference was to Jack Nubbins, twenty yards ahead of the group and still pressing. A promising freshman from the scrub-pine territory north of Orlando, he had been courted by a number of schools until his transcript revealed some troubling deficiencies. When Nubbins arrived at Southeastern on probationary status, he proceeded to tell his other first-year colleagues at Doobey Hall: "Nubbins is the name and I cut the mile in 4:12.3 but I ride a horse better'n that, an' in the fall I hunt wild hog with my grandaddy, sometimes employin' a whepon, sometimes not. Nice ta meetcha."

The other runners, albeit distance men and accustomed to a certain amount of weirdness, judged him loony as a gull and fascinating as all get-out. Cassidy liked him okay, but thought he laughed too loud and got too much mileage out of idioms like "hog-tied" and "gut-shot." Additionally, he appeared to lack a certain . . . *respect*.

"I don't think he is going to be able to restrain himself this morning," Cassidy muttered irritably. Some of the other runners were trying to pick up the pace to catch Nubbins and the group was starting to string out. The unspoken rule against racing had a sanction: those who persisted at it might well find themselves in a death match with an upperclassman.

"You did twenty-seven yesterday, didn't you?" Cassidy said.

"Yup."

"You wouldn't want to come along anyway, would you? Just for grins?"

"Nope."

"That's what I thought. See ya."

"See ya."

NUBBINS HAD BEEN A PRODIGY in high school; he had indeed run the mile in 4:12 and had very nearly broken 9:00 for two miles. These were impressive accomplishments for a schoolboy athlete and gave Nubbins unarguable status among his young peers. A strong runner such as he, unfettered by a sense of unity and left unrestrained, would simply destroy most of his teammates. Soon he would represent to them the pinnacle, the ultimate competitor; he would forever be the ceiling of their accomplishment. If his were a certain kind of personality, he would accept this responsibility with love and great modesty. As long as he was undisputedly their vanquisher, he would laugh and joke with them and pound their backs in ribald camaraderie; then daily on the trails or roads or track, he would casually stomp them into submission. Mizner called it the "Top Dog Syndrome."

Everyone was competitive with his fellows to a certain extent; being bested in a daily workout by one's teammates did not portend well for the time when one went out to take on the rest of the world. But Cassidy was trying to bring the younger runners along without resorting to humbling daily comparisons. He was stronger than they were; he wanted them to know it, but not to dwell on it. There is time, he would tell them; time and time and time. He wanted to impart some of the truths Bruce Denton had taught him, that you don't become a champion by winning a morning workout. The only true way is to marshal the ferocity of your ambition over the course of many days, weeks, months, and (if you could finally come to accept it) years. The Trial of Miles; Miles of Trials. How could he make them understand?

Nubbins was nowhere near a slouch. He was fast and courageous and mentally tough and he had nine state high school titles to prove it. Like all good runners, he gave away nothing. Cassidy knew he had long taken winning for granted, that he was accustomed to looking over at an opponent with a kind of detached pity and then surging off with great style.

The gradual sense of despair Nubbins now felt was a new and discomfiting experience. He had never run with a nonnegotiable shadow before. He picked it up just a tad more, but Quenton Cassidy (his T-shirt read: GAUNT IS BEAUTIFUL) just looked over and smiled back pleasantly.

"You feeling pretty good, Jack?" Cassidy asked on the exhale.

"Not too bad, I reckon." Nubbins tried to grin.

"Good," Cassidy said, as he kicked the pace down about ten seconds a mile. A minute later, just as Nubbins was almost accustomed to the now alarming pace, Cassidy threw in a thirty-two-second 220. They were now all but sprinting along the early morning sidewalk. Nubbins's face was both tight and pale. His expression said that he was a man with a problem.

They flew along at sub-five-minute pace, quite fast enough to startle pedestrians. They blew into the last mile, came upon and passed on either side of a sleepy coed bound for first-period class: reams of biology notes filled the air.

MIZNER TROTTED UP to the front porch steps of Doobey Hall where Cassidy sagged in repose.

"Well," he said, "is he a believer yet?"

"Hell if I know. Jeez, he's a tough little bastard. Next time you take him. Did you see him back there anywhere?"

"Yeah, passed him half a mile back. Said he was turning off to go lift weights at the field house. That what he told you?"

"No, all he said to me was: 'Aaack.'"

"Aaack?"

"Aaack. And then he bent over and grabbed his knees and commenced serious air sucking."

IN THE WORLD OF THE RUNNER, as in the ocean, there is a hierarchy of ferocity. In the sea the swift blue runner is eaten by the slashing barracuda, which is eaten by the awesome mako shark. In track, such relative positions are fixed more or less in black and white and are altered only at great and telling expense. Pride necessarily sprouts and grows; a pride that can only come from relentless kneading of unwilling flesh, painful months of grinding and burning away all that is heavy, all that is strength-

sapping and useless to the body as a projectile. The runner
becomes almost haughty. He looks to those stronger with respect
and fear, to those slower with sympathy or tolerance (they tread
ground he has long since covered). The jettisoning of but a single
second is announced like a birth in the family.

Quenton Cassidy had run one mile in 4:00.3 and despite the
near indifference of the sporting world, four-minute milers are
still very nearly as rare a breed as, say, astronauts. The name
"Cassidy" appeared in the school record books eight separate
times counting the various relays. Though Jack Nubbins was a
talented young runner, Quenton Cassidy had viewed the
Specter; when he reached down through the familiar layers of
gloom and fatigue he generally found more there than a name-
less and transient desire to acquire plastic trophies. He and
Nubbins were not even in the same ballpark.

"GOOD MORNING, Captain Cassidy," called Michael Mobley, the
all-American shot-putter. He surrounded his table as if it were a
toy.

"Good morning, Captain Mobley," Cassidy called back. "Join
you in just a moment." Cassidy had probably started this exaggerated politeness among the tricaptains. He had a helpless
affinity for harmless traditions.

The dining room at Doobey Hall was suggestive of what
might happen if a cargo plane full of raw sirloin were to crash in
Lion Country Safari. Several dozen athletes screamed, laughed,
cajoled, and punched one another in the easy fond intimacy that
sports give to young men in groups and that they would con-
sciously or subconsciously miss for the rest of their lives.

The good-humored pandemonium was considerable as they
consumed caloric numbers more befitting a small town. The relatively thin distance runners ate more than you would expect
(Cassidy loaded his tray with three scrambled eggs, two pan-

cakes, sausage, nearly a quart of milk, and two doughnuts for later). A colossus like Mobley, however, simply ate with a vengeance. With unswerving deliberation and concentration, he sat and *consumed*.

"Got to keep up my strength, right?" he would say. "Otherwise you gotta go to anabolic steroids and I don't want my nuts to shrivel up like peanuts, right?" He laughed like a bass drum.

The weight men were cocky, masculine, and actually fairly gentle; they never needed to bully, such was their looming physical presence. These specimens made their particular way in the world by heaving sixteen-pound iron balls great distances, tossing fiberglass plates out of vision, whipping sharpened aluminum shafts to the horizon. They were the most direct throwbacks to ancient times when such arts were cultivated to bash and puncture the armor of one's enemies; to spill blood from a distance. They were the heavy artillery of old. The confidence of those who do such things well is enormous and needs no bravado for support. They feared only one another.

The distance runners were serene messengers. Gliding along wooded trails and mountain paths, their spiritual ancestors kept their own solitary counsel for long hours while carrying some message the import of which was only one corner of their considerable speculation. They lived within themselves; long ago they did so, and they do today.

There was great unspoken respect between the weight men and the distance runners that was understood but never examined closely. They all dealt in one way or another with the absolute limits of the human body and spirit, but the runners and weight men seemed to somehow share a special understanding, and there were good friendships among them.

The sprinters and jumpers were quite another story. Their art revolved around a single explosive instant during which all was gained or lost. They were, perhaps, the spiritual descendants of the assault troops who leaped trenches and scaled barricades to lead the attack. They were nervous, high-strung, either giddy with success or mired in swamp funk. They were the manic-depressives of the track world. They constantly puffed themselves up with braggadocio, either to bolster their own flagging courage or to intimidate their opponents. The intensity of their competition was ferocious, almost cruel. A high jumper is in the air less than a second and a half. A sprinter's race takes ten seconds. A pole vaulter stands with fiberglass catapult in hand and contemplates his task far longer than the three seconds he struggles in the aspic of space. Cassidy pitied them the intensity of their contests, but at the same time was envious. One would grunt with the enormous effort, elastic muscles responding from years of weight training and explosive exercise, soaring up, up, and turning on an axis of perfect technique (so quick you would miss the beauty of it if you did not know what to look for), an awful moment of hate-filled glaring at the dreaded black-and-white bar—a fragile, shame-bearing obstruction, loathsome to the touch—and then a free fall (throwing your fist with joy and relief) back to earthly cares. Yes, there was something to that, Cassidy would think, particularly on a hot spring day when he had to run fifteen or twenty quarter miles on a sticky track shimmering with heat.

In any event, Cassidy's table companions made for lively dining. He and Mizner, still damp from the shower, finished filling their trays and sat down across from Mobley, who gave the impression of eating with both hands.

"Heard you guys were scalding dogs this morning," Mobley said, without halting the intake.

"Now just why the details of a morning run would be of interest to a member of the gorilla corps is certainly beyond me," said Mizner, who well knew that Mobley reacted to no brash comments. The giant, all six feet six, 265 pounds of him, scarcely stopped chewing. He looked up with an expression that was something less than annoyance.

"Just be sure to keep those little dweebs in line, please, Captain," he told Cassidy, shoveling in half a pancake. He gulped. "We've got a chance to win some big brass at conference this year and your pond birds are gonna have to get their points."

"Pond birds, is it?" said Mizner, pounding his spoon like an impatient child. "Pond birds? I have a good mind to pump up for a couple of months and take your young ass on." The imagery evoked by such a notion caused considerable merriment around the room.

4.

Cross-country

Cassidy's year, a runner's year, was divided into three parts. Fall was cross-country, a season of six-mile races that stretched from the heat of Florida's long Indian summer to the frozen slush of November in the North and West. Winter was the indoor season, a time of exciting races on the little banked wooden tracks in the large cities of the Northeast. Spring and early summer were for what Denton called "real track." During the bleak expanse of fall and winter, however, "real track" was too far off to think about.

Cassidy did not like cross-country; the distance was too long for a miler, he disliked not being able to "feel" the finish line during the race. Six miles seemed interminable to a runner accustomed to the blissful unyielding symmetry of four quarter miles run in nearly sixty seconds each (he never felt the first lap, the second and third were pure hell but over quickly, and the last went by in the giddy excitement of the sprint and the locked-up zombie gait of total oxygen debt).

"What's wrong with cross-country?" Denton asked. Warm-down time was slow luxury, an easy mile of deep, aching satisfaction.

"Some weird people like it, I know that. I'm very aware of that," Cassidy said. A muted glance passed between Denton and Mizner. They had heard this before.

"Six miles . . . ten thousand meters," Cassidy said disgustedly, "over hill and dale out in the middle of nowhere. Spit freezing on your goddamn chin. Five hundred complete wild men in the mud, running up on your heels with long spikes. Oh, I love cross-country, all right. I also like being flayed alive with a rusty straight razor."

"Why, Quenton, you were *county champion* in high school. I saw it in your scrapbook. You had a clipping from the morning paper and a clipping from the evening paper. Don't you remember?" Denton asked seriously. Mizner bit his lip.

"Sticking my tongue in a light socket, that's a lot of fun too," Cassidy said moodily.

"But you *did* win the—"

"Yes, and for your information it was my *mother* who cut out those clippings, you can tell by how neatly they are trimmed. I don't operate that way."

"Quenton Cassidy, *cross-country champion* . . ."

"It was a two-point-five-mile race and the competition was fierce, lads. Several local entries could have been real trouble if the race had only been two and a quarter miles shorter. They were the kind of guys who yell and scream for the first hundred yards, you know, like they are having a good time and all . . ."

"But they couldn't hold the pace, eh?"

"It kills me when they yell and scream like that, or talk back and forth to each other real nonchalant like it's not bothering them at all." Cassidy looked genuinely puzzled.

"But tough cookies nonetheless?" Denton wouldn't let him off the hook.

"To a man." Cassidy grinned at Mizner. "I leaned at the tape and nipped second place by about half a mile. Maybe they sent the wrestling team by accident. Anyway, Palm Beach County is not noted for its cross-country strength."

"Half a mile is what Mize usually gets you by, isn't it?"

Cassidy feigned hurt. "You don't need to rub it in. I *told* you I don't like it. You distance animals can have it. Milers are too fine-tuned to enjoy that pastoral crap."

"So are road runners, race walkers, orienteering nuts, and a bunch of other folks looking to avoid real confrontation," Denton said.

"Right," Mizner said. He liked watching Cassidy having to take it for a while.

"Real confrontation is four laps and a cloud of . . . Tartan dust," Cassidy said.

"That's clever."

"Tartan dust?" Mizner asked.

"Oh yes, that's really clever." Denton shook his head.

"You guys can just blow it out your—"

"Steady, big fellow," Denton said in his mock-deep voice, the Lone Ranger calming old Silver down after a hard day of chasing desperadoes. Cassidy laughed and threw a halfhearted elbow at Denton, who dodged and rolled his eyes.

Coach Benjamin Cornwall was getting into his car when he saw the three of them jostling one another at the door of the field house. Weary from his own work, he never could figure out what it was about a twenty-mile day that made some people so playful.

𝒞

"THREE MORE?" Cassidy asked.

"At least."

He and Mizner did hundred-yard striders in the grass, trying to build up some lactic acid resistance and get the systems moving. They wanted to be well into what some people call "the second wind" before the race started. The runners usually referred to it by the physiologists' term, "homeostasis." Whatever it is called, it entails a good hard warm-up. They had already run three miles at an easy pace.

Dual meets were not at all hectic and Cassidy didn't really mind this miniature version of cross-country. A single team would not usually have enough talent to present much of a challenge, even to Cassidy. Neither he nor Mizner considered this particular Saturday important enough to slack off their training in the slightest. They had both run sixteen miles the day before, a gambit known as "running through" a meet. When you are beaten by an athlete running through, it means you are owned by him body and soul. The Fixed Order will have been established in a most definitive way, to be altered only by some kind of felonious conduct, possibly involving antipersonnel mines.

Bruce Denton ran up from behind them and fell in with their strides. Even at this quick pace his legs moved with a ghostly lack of effort. Runners from the other team stole glances at him. Cassidy thought: the little sons of bitches are experiencing awe.

"You doing your morning?" Mizner asked.

"Yep. Thought I'd come over and watch the fun."

"I hate racing in the morning like this," Cassidy offered.

"There's not a whole lot about this deal you *do* like, is there, sport?" Denton smiled at him.

"Not much, I guess," Cassidy admitted gloomily. "My gut goes crazy . . ."

"Do these guys have any horses?" Denton asked.

"The redheaded fellow," said Mizner, gesturing. "The one so very obviously not looking at us. That's Eammon O'Rork, a genuine imported Irishman. Guess they couldn't afford themselves an African." Mizner was unconsciously mimicking Cassidy.

"Gave you a scare last year indoors, didn't he, sport?" Denton turned to Cassidy.

"'Scare' isn't the word. It was the Mason-Dixon Games in Louisville. The score was, the Kid: four oh three point two; the Irish Upstart: four oh three point two. But it was closer than it sounds."

Denton laughed as they started another strider. O'Rork's freckled face was clouded with concentration as he did his own warm-up. He glanced constantly at his watch, timing it to the minute. They had about eight minutes before assembling for the starting instructions.

O'RORK WAS OLDER than the rest of his team; older and far more mature. His talent and courage had delivered him from the rigors of life in Northern Ireland and he went at distance running with the uncomplicated ardor of the truly hungry. Denton appraised the Irishman's stride as he went by and thought: There is always something behind it, isn't there, fellow? With us and prizefighters, the wounded and the fleet . . .

O'Rork was thinking about Cassidy's cloth-thin victory the previous season. It still rankled him. The American was all right, he supposed, just too blithe a spirit to suit O'Rork. A few weeks after the Louisville meet O'Rork had picked up an intestinal flu and was all but incapacitated during much of the outdoor season. It had been a bad December: a telegram (hanging in a serious-looking plastic envelope on his dormitory-room door) brought the bad news from home. He had sat quietly for five minutes looking at the sad little yellow message, then he pulled on his training shoes and went out to run himself into a blubbering mush in the hills surrounding his Tennessee campus. Then he was in bed for two weeks and really wouldn't have minded dying. Cold Decembers, he thought, watching the carefree American. I have known too many of them.

THEY WERE LESS THAN a half mile from the finish; Cassidy ran slightly behind O'Rork off his left shoulder, eyes fixed on the freckled neck. He was drafting without malice or humor. If O'Rork minded being used in this manner he gave no sign.

Somewhere up ahead Jerry Mizner was sauntering into the finish chute with the more tolerable fatigue of victory on his face. He had employed the simple expedient of running away from everyone. Similarly isolated from the rest of the runners, the two milers bruised each other in the tensionless grind of those who struggle for second place.

Cassidy was in extremis. They had gone through the first mile in 4:37 and Cassidy thought with alarm: *Godamighty that hurt*. The heavy training of the past several weeks had sapped him; when he reached down for an extra surge just to hold pace, he found only a searing strained feeling with which he was intimately familiar: redline city. He was not enjoying his weekend.

Hanging on to O'Rork these past two miles had been possible through a dreary combination of willpower and wishful thinking. Coast, you bastard, Cassidy told himself. Then he put his mind into neutral, locked on to the freckled shoulder, and obtained his mental abstracts: gliding, floating, covering ground. He balked unashamedly at the remarkable discomfort he was living through at the moment. He even thought of tossing it in, not an unusual sentiment, but knew it wouldn't happen. He also kept telling himself that they wouldn't all be this bad because if they were he surely couldn't live with it. He didn't consider himself particularly courageous.

A long path led up the hill through Beta Woods and onto the track for the finish. The hill was steep; it numbed the legs and discouraged fast finishes. O'Rork intentionally worked Cassidy hard on this hill, surgically removing the sting from a kick he remembered quite clearly. Pumping hard, he pulled away. With great distress, Cassidy reeled him back in. This isn't so bad, Cassidy thought, I'm just dying is all. But hang on, asshole, and maybe you can be a hero at the end. The self-loathing was genuine and when he thought about it later it always mystified him.

Every stride now caused him the most profound regret. Spitting fluffy wads of congealed saliva, his thinking soon came only in staccato bursts: two hundred yards . . . keep him near . . . keep him near . . .

Within sight of the finish he could vaguely see Mizner doing a silly bounce and yelling something as Cassidy began to lock up. Andrea would be there somewhere but he didn't see her. A white haze—a normal phenomenon—clouded everything, like looking through the dirty window of a long-abandoned house. Funny how your mind works at the end like this, he thought. The excitement was all outside as he watched quietly from inside his raging skull.

A hundred yards to go, he thought *oh christ* and threw the remainder of what was left into it; now *that* really cost him.

O'Rork burst away from him quickly and won by ten yards.

CASSIDY WAS BENT OVER at the waist, hands on knees, doing a little circle stagger that in other circumstances might have passed for amusing. The other runners were noisily starting to come in. Mizner stood with his arm around Cassidy's waist, providing balance.

"Easy, easy," he said in calm, empathetic tones. Cassidy could not speak; his eyes bulged insanely, breaths came in greedy rasps, and his face was a splotchy violet color.

"Yack!" he said, trying to straighten up. It was too soon; dizziness forced him back to the hands-on-knees death grip, the fetal rest position of the totally done-in runner. The white haze had thickened into a heavy fog; he felt faint but knew his conditioning would protect him from everything but extreme heat. These were the worst few seconds and he understood better than anything else that like the tail fin, the Nehru jacket, and the republic itself, they too would pass. The drained elation, special property and reward of those who have been to the edge and back, would come later. But for now he had awhile longer to hurt.

Andrea, who had never seen such things, stood close by, almost afraid to touch him, hands fluttering around each other and over to his wet singlet. The rasping, dripping, violet-shaded runner studied the moist earth between his spiked toes and seemed unaware of her presence. Was he all right?

"Sure hell, he's all right," Mizner said, surprised by her question. "He's just run himself a *race* is all."

Seeing that Cassidy had his own balance, Mizner went off gaily to check the team scores. Finally straightening up enough to stumble for a few steps, the runner looked at her and said again: "Yack." But this time there was something that could have passed for a smile on his hot face. To her he looked near death— not a mysterious wan passing, but a demise culminating in hot bouts of fever and hallucination, fearful and soul-wrenching. The smile brought her considerable cheer. "Yack?" She smiled back.

"Gee, that was un*com*fortable," he said seriously, as he began to make himself walk; he was unaccustomed to long spikes, one caught, he stumbled as he gripped her hand. "What did you think?"

"I thought you were going to die there for a second. I was afraid."

"Well," he said jovially, "that's the *cross-country biz.*"

Denton stood twenty yards away, chatting with the coaches. But his eyes followed Quenton Cassidy closely.

Half an hour later he gathered up Mizner and Cassidy and the three of them trotted off, laughing, on the eight-mile course to get in some miles for the day.

5

Bowling for Dollars

JERRY MIZNER was an admitted obsessive-compulsive, probably a necessity for a true distance man; his mind adapted well
to the distance runner's daily toil. Cassidy was far more impul-
sive by nature and had to painfully teach himself the record-
keeping, ritualistic, never-miss-a-mile mentality of a dedicated
runner. Mizner and Denton, like Jim Ryun or Gerry Lindgren,
were natural runners who had never even attempted other
sports seriously. Cassidy had good speed, and like Peter Snell
had done well in other sports before concentrating on middle
distances. At times he felt like a spiritual interloper with the
other two; occasionally he was actually jealous of the way they
casually handled the workload. Slowly, for survival's sake, he
learned the lifestyle of the compulsive personality. But when he
occasionally wavered, Mizner felt sorry for him and tried to help

him through the bouts of blue funk and strange behavior. Cassidy would say:

"The Kid is largely unhappy."

"There there."

"Got caught in the rain and muh green stamps got all plastered to muh Sweet'N Low."

"It'll be okay . . ."

"Bet muh money on the bob-tail nag . . ."

The friction caused by superimposing alien psychological traits on his own personality occasionally burst forth in interesting manifestations: Cassidy arranging a quadruple moon shot (the famous Four Way Pressed Ham) out of the tailgate of a duly licensed state vehicle; Cassidy presenting a series of unauthorized awards at the cross-country banquet in mixed company (" . . . and now a very special presentation, the Zazu Pitts Memorial Plaque to the runner who most infrequently committed flatus on the morning run . . ."); Cassidy, as Nubbins put it one night in bewilderment, "just plain walkin' around *talkin'* funny."

Whatever outward form his inner disquietudes took, his odd energies held Doobey Hall like a spell. In this tiny society where the extreme was commonplace, Cassidy's mystique affected everyone. He was often sought out for counsel and his apparent reluctance to render it only added to his aura. His opinion was solicited on matters scholastic, financial, romantic, and mechanical, though he disavowed expertise in all these areas.

He had the gifted athlete's innate sense of timing, a sense of providence, of fantasy, an intuition into the art of the Proper Moment, where the escape velocity of frivolous lunacy triumphs over the mean gravity of everyday life.

By way of example, the doldrums of summer were approaching at the end of his junior year when Cassidy, bored with the hot, ennui-stilled Sunday lunch, posed a general question to the drowsy dining room: "I wonder if Spider can jump over a Volkswagen."

Spider Gordon looked up sleepily from his vegetable soup.

"Of course he can jump over a Volkswagen," said the giant Mobley, his mouth full as usual. "You ought to know that."

"Yes. Yes, of course he can. Spider can easily jump over a Volkswagen," Cassidy said.

Mumbling, everyone turned back to the unexciting lunch, clearly disappointed. What had gotten into Cassidy?

"The *real* question," Cassidy continued after a proper pause, "the real question *here* is whether Spider can jump over *two* Volkswagens!"

The philosophical extensions of this problem became quickly evident and the dining room emptied like a barroom shooting. The neighborhood was scoured for a certain make of foreign car and the entire affair went down in Doobey Hall folklore as "The Day Spider Gordon Busted His Ass on the Fourth Volkswagen."

New members of the team, freshmen or transfer students, were given no special warning about Cassidy. They found out, as everyone else did, in the best way they could.

"Gentlemen," Cassidy would say, rising at dinner and tapping his glass for silence, "we have got to have a plan. We must have a plan even if it is *wrong*." There would come scattered, polite applause.

Chairs scraped as everyone turned their attention to Cassidy's table. Some veterans muttered approval at these odd sentiments while the new guys looked around in stark confusion. After waiting for the buzz to die down, Cassidy continued:

"I realize World Team Bowling is a relatively new concept. But, gentlemen"—a small chuckle here—"as our attendance figures indicate, it is a concept . . . *whose time has come!*" Cheers from the veterans, new guys aghast.

"Now, we have made some mistakes. No one denies that." Negative mumbling; certainly no one was going to deny that. "When our Eye-talian all-star here, Jerry Mizerelli, split his pants on network teevee going for that spare in the sixth frame against Akron, well, gentlemen, it was a bleak moment for our fledgling organization as well as for sports in general. Certainly no one is faulting Jerry for that one, but I'll tell you that all of us, players and management alike, were keeping our fingers crossed. All of us except Jerry, of course, who was doing a medium-slow crab walk with a new Brunswick double ball bag jammed in his crotch . . ."

Well, it was just old crazy Cassidy of course, and maybe the moon was full or something. But he had eaten their bread and salt (and was always walking over exhausted from his race to inquire just how *was* the pole vault going anyway?) and to put it simply he could get away with just about anything with them.

At times he swiveled the spotlight and its harsh glare fell on those not quite so ready for wholesale craziness; it was in this way Mizner had been "discovered." As a new distance man, Mizner had sat around with a dour expression through his first of Cassidy's Bowling Banquets, and had generally been marked off as an old maid until Cassidy suddenly presented him with some mythical honor one night. Mizner stood timidly as Cassidy handed him a Dr Pepper can fashioned into a ridiculous trophy with a scrap of tinfoil. The new runner stared with wide eyes at the bemused, expectant faces around the room. He cleared his throat. A few veterans looked at one another; this was going to be good.

"I, uh, would like to thank Mr. Cassadamius for this here award and I'd like to say something else while I'm standing here. You know, I wasn't really nobody at all when Mr. Cassadamius found me in that little three-lane alley in Pittsburgh. Sure, I mean, I was a local hotshot and all, rolling 210, 215, and just, you know, getting along. But I wasn't no serious contender is what I'm trying to tell ya. Never made the cut or nothin' like that. And then one day Mr. Cassadamius comes in and he watches me roll a few frames, no more'n that, just a few frames, and then he comes over big as day and says, 'Son,' he says, 'Son, if you get rid of that limp wrist of yours and learn to come *over* the ball on your follow-through, you just might knock yourself over a few a' them pins.' I mark that as the turnin' point in my career which has led me to the point at which I am at today." He started to sit down, changed his mind and stood back up, clearing his throat.

"That, uh, and going to the twenty-five-pound composite ball. Thank you."

They sat stunned for several seconds, finally breaking into rowdy applause that quickly became a standing ovation. Mizner looked around the room with a faint smile on his dark face, making little bows with his head.

Cassidy, sitting across from him all moony-eyed, fell smack in love.

6.
Bruce Denton

QUENTON CASSIDY would have thought it amusing had someone called him a great runner. He wasn't even the best in
the neighborhood. Nor was Jerry Mizner, who could claim all-
American honors at the six-mile distance. It wasn't even close:
the best runner around Kernsville was Bruce Denton, a methodical, dryly humorous doctoral candidate in botany. While both
younger runners were formidable talents in collegiate circles,
Denton's place in the hierarchy of distance running was lofty and
secure. The others held him in secret awe and reported his words
to comrades with the solemnity of one reading from the Dead
Sea Scrolls: "Well, now, Denton says you should warm-down like
blah blah . . ." Such pronouncements could halt the most vocifer-
ous arguments.

As an undergraduate at a small school in Ohio, Denton had

been a good but not spectacular performer, running the mile in 4:08. But as with many runners he began to improve with age. He moved to Florida and took up graduate studies at Southeastern, where he began training again with a scientifically precise vengeance. On the altar of Consistency he offered up no less than two portions of his life per day, seven days a week, fifty-two weeks a year. His neatly filled calendar diary told no lies and the symbolism of the unmissed workout became ritualistic to him, taking on an importance in his life he did not like to admit, even to himself.

On a rainy day in November he was so sick with the flu that his wife, Jeannie, felt constrained to stay home from work to look after him. He threw up regularly and had diarrhea so badly his stomach muscles began cramping. Nonetheless, he arose and ran two eerie miles at a stumbling pace, pale and shivering the whole way. His wife was aghast. Again in the afternoon he repeated the process, this time nearly fainting as he staggered back into the apartment. Dr. Stavius—whose claim to fame was that he had once punctured a blister on the foot of Roger Bannister—stormed into Denton's sickroom and pronounced him a madman.

"What crazy?" Denton asked, trying to make his parched lips form a smile. "After today I'm sixteen miles behind for the week."

Over the course of several years at Southeastern, as Denton's reputation grew, a number of undergraduate runners decided they would train with him, thinking to pick up on the Secret. A new man would show up the first day expecting all manner of horrific exertion, and would be stunned and giddy to find he could so easily make it through one of Denton's calendar days. Showing up the second morning at 6:30 he would be of good cheer, perhaps trying to imagine how he would handle the pressure of his inevitable fame. That day would also go well enough, but he would begin to notice something peculiar. There was no letup. The tempo was always moderate but steady. If a new guy decided to pick up the pace, that's where it stayed, whether he finished with the group or not. You showed off at your peril.

On the third day (assuming the new man made it that far) his outlook would begin to darken. For one thing, he was getting very, very tired. No particular day wore him out, but the accumulation of steady mileage began to take its toll. He never quite recovered fully between workouts and soon found himself walking around in a more or less constant state of fatigue-depression, a phase Denton called "breaking down." The new runner would find it more tedious than he could bear. The awful truth would begin to dawn on him: there was no Secret! His days would have to be spent in exactly this manner, give or take a mile or two, for longer than he cared to think about, if he really wanted to see the olive wreath up close. It would simply be the most difficult, heartrending process he would endure in the course of his life.

At that point most of them would drift away. They would search within themselves somewhere along a dusty ten-mile trail or during the bad part of a really gut-churning 440 on the track, and find some key element missing. Sheepishly they would begin to miss workouts, then stop showing up altogether. They would convince themselves: there must be another way, there *has* to be. The attrition rate was nearly a hundred percent.

Only Cassidy and Mizner made it through the process and finally accepted the Trial of Miles. When Denton saw that they were different, he opened up to them and they discovered for the first time that the silently gliding machine at their sides all those months actually had a personality. Accustomed as they were to the flamboyance of their teammates, they were amused by Denton's penchant for understatement. Once, when he returned from the large international road race at Springbank, Canada, they gathered around his locker, waiting for details. Well, they wanted to know, how did it go?

"Not too badly, I guess," said Denton, dressing in his quick, methodical way. "I got in a token mile in the morning and then ran a few after the race so the week's total won't suffer too much. Jogged around the Atlanta airport too." He added the last thoughtfully, scratching his chin.

"Well, goddamn, Bruce, all the Europeans are usually there, Aussies, even some Africans. Who the hell won?" Cassidy was impatient.

"Oh, I won it," Denton said breezily, apparently still thinking about the coup of getting a couple of extra miles at the airport.

"Christ, you won it! Ron Hill, Dave Bedford, Frank Shorter, all those guys usually—"

"Yeah . . ." Denton said, pausing in the middle of tying his shoelace as if remembering something pleasant from his childhood. "Nicest bunch of guys you'd ever want to meet."

WHEN DURING HIS FIRST POSTGRADUATE YEAR Denton came from relative obscurity to run 27:10 for six miles at the Drake Relays, knowledgeable distance buffs were mildly surprised that such an undistinguished performer could run an international-caliber race out of the blue. However unlikely it seemed in retrospect, at the time the phrase "flash in the pan" was bandied about. There are scoffers, it seems, in every field. Later that spring when Denton made the U.S. Olympic team, nearly everyone professed surprise. Everyone except Dr. Stavius and a promising young miler named Quenton Cassidy, who watched the U.S. trials on television. True to form, Denton powered across the finish line in the 5000 meters and simply jogged past the cameras over to his sweats and departed the stadium. Everyone had ignored him for so long, it seemed to Cassidy a delicious gesture.

Now two years after that Olympiad, though they had survived the Trial of Miles and knew his "Secret," and though they were championship collegiate runners, Cassidy and Mizner knew better than anyone that Denton played the game on an entirely different level. He was unencumbered by such things as team standings, dual meets, conference titles; as a graduate student he ran for himself (nominally for the Southeastern University "Track Club," of which he was the sole member). His fare was paid to large meets all over the country by promoters who wanted his name for their posters. During the indoor season he would likely be found in nearly any large city in the country on a given weekend, running either a two-mile (which he called a "deuce") or a three-mile race.

He knew or had run against most of the top runners in the world; he had raced Ron Clarke on the grass in Australia (winning with a big kick); he had suffered through a high-altitude two-mile against the smiling, fierce Kip Keino (losing to a big kick). He had spent several weeks in Eugene with *The Pre,* listening thoughtfully to the Bowerman/Dellinger theorems (tempering his awe with miler Roscoe Divine's confession that he snuck out and ran extra workouts when the assigned ones were too easy). He had listened to Gerry Lindgren say "bad berries" about three thousand times during a hot twenty-miler outside Spokane. He had had a long, pleasant argument with Kenny Moore as to the real value of the Mileage Ethic as opposed to the hard/easy theory, which ended when he told the great marathoner: "You may not *believe* in mileage, but you sure as hell *run* mileage."

There was little wonder Bruce Denton had more quiet confidence than Cassidy or Mizner in the distance runner's little rigid hierarchy of black-and-white numbers, and little wonder why they held him in awe. In his apartment there was an overburdened second bedroom that served as a guest room, study, and trophy room. In the corner was an ancient filing cabinet with locking drawers. In the bottom drawer, the only one that still locked, was a flat oblong leather box.

In that box was an Olympic gold medal.

7.

Andrea

"I'M IN LOVE with her, I tell you," Cassidy said.

"You don't even know her."

"I don't care. If I knew her it might spoil it. Did you see her little forehead, how it was all wrinkled and sweaty?"

"Come on . . ."

"She was concentrating on her *pace* fer chrissakes . . ."

"Awww . . ."

This was how it all began, back at the very start of the school year. The scrap of red yarn she carelessly tied her hair up with might have had something to do with it. Or perhaps it was the *very* sincere look on her face as they trundled by her on the warm-up course that day. Even Mizner commented on how pretty she was.

The typical fetching Southeastern University coed was a

lovely pharmacist's daughter with a hard little body, dairymaid complexion, and the soul of a robber baron. Cassidy had no idea what made Andrea so different, but he could sense that she had somehow survived twenty years as an attractive female in the republic without having had her mind reamed out by mama, the Junior League, or Helen Gurley Brown.

Several days later on the three-mile warm-up they saw her again.

"Try to smooth it out a little," Cassidy suggested as they passed. He demonstrated with an exaggerated version of the classical running stride (a stride that he did not use himself when the chips were down).

She looked up, her damp forehead wrinkled with concentration, and stared at Cassidy as if he were some aquatic parasite that had attached itself to her ankle while she was wading in a creek. Cassidy nearly swooned.

"You're crazy," Mizner told him.

"She appreciated the advice," Cassidy decided.

"She thinks you're crazy too."

"How do you figure?"

"What would you do if some guy out of the blue just up and starts critiquing your stride?"

"Challenge him to a race."

"If his T-shirt said PITTSBURGH HOLY ROLLERS and he started prancing around like this . . . you'd think he was crazy too. And you'd be right."

"Mize, the girl was clearly grateful. She appreciated the advice," Cassidy repeated, troubled.

"The *girl*,"—Mizner was annoyed—"has a gimpy leg. I saw it yesterday when she was stretching up at the track. She probably not only didn't appreciate the advice, she probably thinks you're an asshole."

"Oh."

ℒ

BUT GIVING UP QUICKLY was not in Quenton Cassidy's nature. A week later he saw her at the Gay Nineties, a rather unfortunately named and remarkably heterosexual tavern. Her blond hair was down, but there was no mistaking her. Her white cotton blouse made her thin arms look very tanned and for some reason that sight of her made his heart hurt. He waited around until her two girlfriends got up to play foosball, then made his slew-footed entrance. She saw him coming.

"Well, well. The coach," she said. It was only faintly sarcastic. She even smiled a little, he thought.

"Ah yes, well, I . . ." He spilled a trickle of beer as he started to make some expansive gesture. Idiotically, he began licking foam off his wrist.

"Don't do that," she said.

"Right. Uh, look, I'm sorry if I—"

"That's all right. I was a little annoyed, but then I figured you might have taken a class or something and maybe even knew what you were talking about."

"Not really," he said happily, sliding into the booth across from her. "But I know a bunch of guys who are really good."

"Are you on the track team or something?"

"Yes, indeed," he said, feeling slightly loony watching her green flame eyes in the pale tavern light.

"Oh my. What event do you do?"

"Decathlon," he said.

"Really?" she asked. "How far do you throw it?"

THEY DRIFTED. Dappled by the hard cypress shadows, out into the burning September sun, they drifted. In one of those pleasant cool eddies life sometimes affords the young in fall or spring, they drifted, quite unaware of the not-so-far-off rattle of bones . . .

"I didn't ask to go see the movie," she said. "I thought the book was sophomoric. Baroque and sophomoric. The movie was your idea."

"It was my fault. But your friends were just asking—"

"My friends think *Love Story* is the finest literature to come down the pike since . . . *The Prophet*. You should have eased up on them. Someday they will be producing babies and not causing anyone any trouble at all."

"All I meant was that such cornpone has a way of co-opting real life. I mean, it's fun to talk snazzy and run around and play in the snow with *yur girl,* for chrissakes, but I don't know if I'll ever be able to throw a dog a Frisbee without thinking I should be in slow motion or something."

"Tear ducts raped. 'I resent having my tear ducts raped' I believe is what you said."

"Awww."

"And were following up with something about the teensy-weensy sexual members of dope-crazed screenwriters or something . . ."

"Well . . ."

"Mary Ellen Conastee was close to having a stroke. She's a harmless girl, Quenton. You're going to have to break in a little slower with some people."

He looked over and gave her what he thought of as his pixie grin.

"Don't give me that pixie-grin crap," she told him.

They drifted. Cassidy was plopped without grace in his inner tube, his white bottom now thoroughly chilled by the icy waters of the Ichetucknee River. Andrea somehow accomplished a similar position without the same loss of dignity: on her it looked sultry. When she leaned back to take the sun he looked carefully at the two brown legs draped over the edge of her tube, but could hardly detect the difference between them that would forever put a little catch in her walk.

Of course there would be something like that; he lacked

interest in the perfect item. Quenton Cassidy, unmoved by kittens, sonnets, and sunsets, was nonetheless given to tragic flaws.

IN ORDER TO ARRANGE THIS DAY of perfect drifting, an entirely traditional local pastime, he and Mizner—now floating up ahead with his date—had arisen at 7:30 and run seventeen miles. It was the only way they could spend their day in the sweet haze of Boone's Farm apple wine and still appease the great white Calendar God whose slighted or empty squares would surely turn up someday to torment the guilt-ridden runner. They went through such contortions occasionally to prove to themselves that their lives didn't have to be so abnormal, but the process usually just ended up accentuating the fact. There were several ways it could be done. If they were going to the beach, they might put it off and run when they got there, but contrary to popular opinion, beach running is only jolly fun for the first five miles or so. After that, the cute little waves become redundant, the sand reflects the sun up into the eyes blindingly, grains of sand slip annoyingly into the heel of the shoe or flip up on the back of the leg. Fifteen hot miles on a long, flat beach sounds like good sport only to those who haven't actually done it. Also, the ocean is too infinite; the run seems as if it will never end.

They could always put training off until they got back in the evening, but that just made things worse. No beer! None of the sticky wine! Their friends would slyly try to tempt them, see if they really took all that training stuff seriously. It was too much to ask. Better to get it all over with and then be able to enjoy the day like any other citizen.

Though he hated running long in the morning more than anything he could think of, Cassidy was ecstatic to have his whole day's training behind him. The oversized tubes floated along on the gin-clear river, meandering slowly under the spooky cypress stands and pleasantly out into splotches of sun. Even though it was Florida, it was *north* Florida and, as winter approached, tubing would be forgotten until spring.

Cassidy paddled over awkwardly to Andrea's tube and invited her to double up. Flirting with disaster for several seconds, she finally accomplished the maneuver.

"Next time you do the transfer at sea, please," she said. Her warmth beside him was searing; she smelled of summer, youth, Sea & Ski, and moist, slightly sweet sex. Clearly edible. His head spun from the wine and sun. Muscles along the top of his thighs trembled from his morning exertion. In a month or so he knew they would carry him screaming around the track. He had the power.

"Ouch!" she said. "What's that all about?"

8

Dick Doobey

THE HEAD FOOTBALL COACH pushed the sweaty baseball cap back on his bristly crew-cut head, leaned way back in his $1,495 Execu-Kliner, plopped his ripple-soled coaching shoes up on his gigantic gleaming desk and wondered what in the world was becoming of him.

With mournful pride he surveyed the wide expanse of lush maroon and silver carpeting that displayed in the very center a custom-woven and very savage-looking Daryl the Swamp Dawg; the office was so large as to invite speculation as to which indoor sports might be accommodated.

The Rotarians had been most unkind. Whereas several years ago he would have been treated with the unbridled respect and admiration due a United States senator or even a big-money media evangelist, this day's luncheon had been laced with a certain ill-concealed nastiness that now knitted Dick Doobey's brow like a ten-dollar pot holder.

L. T. Doaches, owner of the Fat Boy's Pit Barbecue off Interstate 75, had posed the question: since Doobey's first three years had allegedly been "rebuilding" years for the ol' Swamp Dawgs, and keeping in mind certain early and somewhat rash predictions, in retrospect how did the coach view this past season's 4-6 record? As L.T. put it: "I mean, are we gonna start rebuilding again without seein' what it was we got ourseffs built the last time?"

It was a mouthful of a question, L.T. having obviously practiced it some, but he delivered it without a flaw and, to the affirmative grumbles and guffaws of the group, replaced his pear-shaped bottom on the Holiday Inn folding chair, Dick Doobey meanwhile discerning all he wanted to know about the general Rotarian mood.

A little surprised by the brewing hostility, he babbled something about some real fine junior college transfers, some red-shirts who would be "a real great help to us out there next year," and a few other favorite mouth-worn Doobey maxims. Kernsville cynics suspected that the NCAA held yearly seminars for the purpose of allowing football coaches to swap these fluffs of wisdom back and forth. Doobey's favorite was: "In order to win you've got to avoid losing first." Things like that.

The same material that at one time would have at least won nodding approval now netted him a few muffled coughs. He was dying up there with a live mike and a glass of watery iced tea. He tried to tell some funny anecdotes, generally racially tinged, mangled one-liners uttered by some player or another, the punch line of which inevitably began: "Well, gosh, Coach . . ."

As a last resort he told some of his My Daddy Used to Say chestnuts that always won chuckles of nostalgia for the old man if not appreciation for his fumbling offspring. Nothing worked. Finally, one sportswriter, a short Jewish fellow Doobey disliked intensely, asked Doobey's opinion of the DUMP DICK DOOBEY bumper stickers that were showing up on cars in and around Kernsville.

Doobey cleared his throat. "Well, now, there has always been dissident elements, you see, in our American System, and while these people may think they are doing the right thing, and while they are certainly entitled to their opinion, you see, such disloyalty to the program can only . . ."

This tack also netted him little in the way of positive Rotarian feedback. It was becoming painfully obvious to him that many of these very Rotarians were either among the "dissident elements" or were sympathetic to them.

Dick Doobey was discovering that a football coach in a small Southern town walks upon water only if he is either "rebuilding" or else whaling tar out of Ole Miss. There is no middle ground called "Holding Your Own." And you can sell the "rebuilding" excuse only so long before you find your career folding up like a ten-year-old road map. Uprisings are fomented; Rotarians go on cautious rampages; and—oh, the infamy!—the very bumpers of automobiles call for your destruction.

DICK DOOBEY took his feet off the desk and pressed the intercom.

"Mary Lou, come on in here a minute, willya, hon?" His mind reeled with daring, if half-baked, strategems. Mary Lou, hoping for hanky-panky, bounced in, miniskirted and primed for action; she sported an alarming beehive hairdo.

"Shall I get the key to the whirlpool?" she asked coyly.

"Uh, not now, hon. I need you to take something down for me." Frowning slightly, she left to get her steno pad.

"This will be a memo to all coaches from Dick Doobey as Athletic Director, not head football coach. You, ah, don't need to write all that down, hon, I mean word for word and all. Like when I said 'not head football coach' you didn't need to write 'not head . . .' Well, you know what to put." Her shoulders sagged impatiently. *What an incredible mind,* she thought. They went through something like this nearly every time.

Doobey waited self-consciously for a few moments as if to allow his words to fall from the air so he could start fresh.

"Ahem. New Rules on Hair Groomin' and Dress, uh, Procedures for Southeastern University Athletes . . ."

9.

An Afternoon

THE RUNNERS CIRCLED the big grass field in a slow, prancing jog, their shirtless bodies gleaming with sweat. As they trotted by Ben Cornwall, they all looked up at him almost simultaneously. Their rasping and coughing grew louder as they approached.

"One thirty-eight. Two to go, guys," the coach told them. They immediately lowered their heads and continued jogging. They were on their rest interval, respite in the acid storm.

Cornwall walked back across the field to catch the next 660 on his split-timer. A 330 jog wasn't much recovery time and he could tell by the strain on their faces that they were working hard. The last two would be quicker perhaps but Cassidy and Mizner had made sure the first six were evenly paced and fast. Cornwall studied his two star runners as he crossed the field to the opposite post. They looked less distraught than the rest, but not by much. Cassidy was saying something to Mizner, who replied with a thin smile. Cornwall couldn't hear it, of course, and wouldn't have understood if he had. The conversation, between gasps, went like this:

"There must be some mistake," Cassidy said. "I have not yet attained that sense of euphoria commonly reported by runners."

"You are speaking no doubt of the fabled 'third wind.'"

"I'm not sure. I haven't read *Runner's World* lately so I don't know what they are calling it this month."

When they reached the post Cornwall clicked the expensive timer and studied with admiration the easy power of the runners flowing into their long strides. The head track coach, oddly enough, didn't know a great deal about distance running (Cassidy and Mizner were constantly—though very unobtrusively— amending his workouts), having been a javelin man in college.

But Cornwall understood that the half milers, milers, and true distance men were the heart of a track team. They could run everything from the mile relay on up. It was imperative that he pay attention to their training.

He had learned very early, though, that the milers and distance men were like seeds: the good ones, given minimum care, just grew on their own. He had only a casual jogger's appreciation for their training—he knew from his own days of conditioning that what they were doing before his eyes was far beyond his ken—and he knew the daily grind took its toll. The attrition rate was startling. Even the most promising runners, disheartened by injuries or poor performances, would sometimes leave their scholarships on his desk. He never tried to talk them out of it; he knew that once they lost it, it was gone for good.

Now as he watched across the big field, the runners entered the far turn with Cassidy and Mizner still leading. Up close their breathing would make a considerable racket, but from here they appeared to be gliding along without effort. From the middle of the pack a shorter runner moved up to their shoulders. Without even having to squint, Cornwall knew it would be Nubbins. If they didn't break him, Cornwall thought, that Nubbins might turn out to be something after all.

Entering the far straight, Cassidy and Mizner picked up the pace slightly and only Nubbins hung on with them. They seemed to sense his presence, but showed no outward sign of it. In an interval workout there was no objection to a hard finish so long as the early running had been even and taxing. Dogging in the early stages in order to shine later on was considered antisocial behavior. Cassidy saved his fiercest workout kick for such occasions.

But Nubbins had been conscientious and was now making a bid for status. He knew very well Cornwall was watching closely. Cassidy slackened somewhat and Nubbins went by, pulling up to Mizner as they came out of the turn. But when the freshman bore down in the last straight and tried to pull away, Mizner matched him stride for stride. Cornwall smiled as he clicked the split-timer for them. He looked down at the watch and thought: *Jesus.* They had run 1:28. Nubbins looked entirely washed out, a face without hope or humor, but he kept on jogging. Cassidy caught up to Mizner and they trotted along without speaking. Cornwall still did not understand that pairing; they were so different. Cassidy was breezy, almost lighthearted for a runner; Mizner was studious and serene. But they were identical in one respect: the haunted cast of their eyes as they entered a gun lap was exactly the same. The coach walked back across the field, still studying Cassidy and Mizner jogging through their rest interval. Those two, he thought. I'll never get another pair like them. Just read the watch for them, see they get fed, get them their plane tickets, and keep them in shoes—no small expense—and they'll go out and win everything in sight.

They were chugging up to him now, looking up from their despondent jog with the same expectant expression. It always amused him how interested they were in the numbers, no matter how exhausted; it was the first thing they wanted to know after a race, even from the depths of their distress.

"Leaders 1:28, Cass 1:29.5, everyone else hit at about 1:33. Last one, fellows." The runners were jogging especially slowly now; this was the way they always did it. Everyone would want to be as fresh as possible for the last one in order to end on an upbeat.

Actually, they would still be out of breath when they started the last one, and Cornwall thought again how surprising it was that after the first several intervals they looked as bad as they would get. The rest seemed to take no more out of them, though he knew each one had to be more difficult than the one before. But then they blew into the last one like they couldn't think of a better way to end the day. They were a strange crowd, runners, Cornwall thought. They were strange back in his track days and they were still strange.

They finally arrived at the starting post with their mincing little steps and with a deep gasp leaned into the last one as Cornwall clicked the watch. They flew into the first turn and Cornwall smiled again. Cassidy was already ten yards in front. By the time they were out of the turn and into the far straight, he was twenty-five yards ahead and still telescoping away. Mizner smoothly led the rest of the pack. Around the final turn and into the straightaway Cassidy powered on with crisp businesslike strides. There was a lift in his stride and from his expression Cornwall could tell he was serious. Forty yards in front Cassidy flashed by the post and Cornwall flicked the watch at him in that strange little "gotcha" affectation of earnest timers everywhere. The coach let out a little grunt as he glanced briefly at the watch before catching the others on the second sweeping hand. Cassidy did not keep jogging as before, but curved back in a parabola of expectation.

"Whyn't you get your ass in gear, Cassidy?" the coach asked.

Cassidy was still gasping, and unamused.

"C'mon. Coach. What. Was it?"

"You think I don't know when you guys are loafing?"

Cassidy rolled his eyes at that, but stood panting, hands on hips. Let him have his fun.

"You had 1:24.6." The coach smiled. "Everyone else was right about 1:29." Cassidy nodded, satisfied, and started to jog off toward Bruce Denton, who stood wringing wet, watching from the side of the field.

"That's about right," Cassidy called back. "Last year would have been 1:26 something about this time." Cornwall knew how accurate his training records were and that Cassidy wasn't guessing.

"You might even do some good in cross-country pretty soon, you keep this up," the coach called out to him. He knew it was a sore point. Mizner had caught up to the other pair as they headed off for the one-mile warm-down course.

"Right," Cassidy called back, "and I might run the hundred in nine flat and play wide receiver for the Dolphins."

CASSIDY SLUMPED ON THE BENCH, draped immodestly with a towel, more or less savoring the deep itchy ache of the last 660 and apparently studying his toes with great interest. He would be losing another nail soon. *Ugliest feet in the world,* he thought, next to Denton's. He ran his hand up and down his left Achilles tendon. Very tender; better pay attention to it and back off if it gets any worse. Maybe ice it. The old Injury Evasion Fandango. Did it ever end?

The afternoon workout had cost him seven pounds. He longed for cooler weather. In the shower Denton laughed: "It's the lean wolf that leads the pack."

"If I am captured in Indochina," Cassidy told him, "I will not last out the night in a bamboo cage."

"Just walk out between the bars," Denton had suggested.

The older runner had been impressed with the 660 workout, but mildly disapproved of doing hard intervals so early in the year. He had settled for a twelve-mile run himself.

"It's easy for you to criticize," Cassidy said, still slumping on the bench while Denton dressed quickly. "You won't be doing the old one-mile run on some little eleven-lap roller-derby track in a few weeks. I need me some *get-down* speed out there."

"When did you turn into a black sprinter?" Mizner asked, "What's this 'get-down' stuff?"

"He's a miler person, you see," Denton said, "and he's explaining about how it's dog eat dog out there. Right, sport?"

Into the steamy and subdued postworkout atmosphere charged Daniel Hayes Ingram, a student trainer whose round face was a sad pink-and-white topographical map of adolescence. In high school Ingram had secured a place on the track team and set about accomplishing his lifelong goal: a five-minute mile. Having failed—by 3.4 seconds—he learned how to tape ankles and apply ice packs and was thus spared eternal exile from that intimate neutral world where the sounds were of rushing water, rough laughter, and the click-clack of brittle spikes on tiled floors. Substitute gratification does not vent completely the deeper yearnings, however, and Danny Ingram was known as a highly excitable person. He now clucked and sputtered with such energy as to gather a small crowd. If the news was not of interest, they would at least get to watch a trainer go mad.

"They got Walton!" Ingram gasped for the third time. The track men looked at one another.

"*John Walton, you idiots! They got John Walton!*" Ingram was exasperated by their blank stares. They knew *who* he was talking about, but could not get the context. They calmed him with abuse and made him begin slowly. He had their interest now and they were going to get to the bottom of this.

"I was just in Cornwall's office . . ."—he took a deep breath—

"and the telegram just came in from the New Zealand travel committee. Walton has agreed to run in the Southeastern University Relays this spring! He's on tour then and had the weekend open. Holy Jesus Christ, John Walton running here! Won't that just be something else now? Can you imagine what he'll do to all these yokels around here when he . . ."

It was a particularly awkward thing to say, for as the import of the news had finally come across, the others had turned almost as a man to see what kind of reaction would issue from the distance runners' corner, where Cassidy and Denton sat watching them with great interest.

"Well, I didn't mean you of course, Cass, uh . . ." But the trainer was clearly into his own pit and his clambering around only brought more debris down upon himself. It was very quiet. Big fans in the roof beat at the hot air.

"Who did you say was coming to the relays, Danny?" Cassidy asked.

"Uh, Walton, John Walton, the miler from New—"

"John Walton? Is he supposed to be pretty good?" Cassidy maintained a countenance of innocent curiosity. Denton turned slightly and coughed.

"Yeah, well, he's *only* run 3:49 and all . . ." Some of the others were snickering but Danny had a very high embarrassment threshold. "Say, Cass"—he was all curiosity now—"how do you think you'll, uh, handle, you know, the . . . situation?"

Cassidy pondered. He looked at the ceiling and sphincterized his lips. Then his face lit up: inspiration!

"I think what I would do would be to hang right with him, see . . ."

"Yeah, well . . ."

"Check him out *real* close, like for a couple of laps. Make *him* take the initiative, see, make *him* run *my* race, see . . ." Denton was leaning against his locker, biting on a towel.

"But *John Walton*, I mean, when he—"

"Then going into the last lap, I'll be right on his tail, see, all the way into the last turn . . ."

"But they say his kick—"

"Then I'll take a shortcut across the infield, sprint down the pole vault runway, and lean at the tape. Works every time."

The assemblage dispersed in what might be called a good mood, but there was an eeriness in the air. Some names were uttered with reverence in that tiled sanctum and John Walton's was one of them. Surely Bruce Denton's name was accorded similar respect in other locker rooms around the world, but there was always something even more mysterious and exotic about those far-off heroes, rarely seen in person, whose feats were frozen for all time in irrefutable black-and-white numerals. Walton's aura, as the first human being to run the mile under 3:50, was that of almost total invincibility. To the public he may have been just one more in a long line of champions, but to those whose own numerals gave credentials of insight, Walton's name brought with it an unpleasant chill. A 3:55-miler would understand it better than a 4:05-miler. Walton was the best there was, but he was only an image to most of them. And now that he was to be viewed in person—take the form of flesh and blood—no one knew quite what to think.

Bruce Denton was an Olympian. He was accustomed to unstable atmospheres where heady names such as Walton's were bandied about like so many harmless acquaintances, but these undergraduates clearly were not, despite their best efforts to act nonchalant.

"Aw, he pulls on his shorts the same way we do," said one of the freshmen. But it didn't dispel Walton's ghost in the least.

"That's right." Denton chuckled. "Except he pulls *his* shorts up over legs that can run a mile in three minutes and forty-nine seconds."

Some of them laughed as they finished dressing, but there was no further discussion. Cassidy still sat on the bench, towel draped across his middle, too weary even to clothe himself. He looked up at Denton and smiled. His 660 workout didn't seem like such hot stuff anymore.

An awesome creature—up until recently more myth than mortal—was to assume human form and cross oceans to perform his magic right on the same track that held their sweat. In doing so he would necessarily devastate those who sought to test his power. That this force would be inexorably brought to bear upon one they all knew, one they had come to respect for his own prowess, made everyone at the same time uneasy and strangely elated. They had rarely seen Quenton Cassidy lose a mile race, did not *want* to see him lose, yet the inevitability of the prospect was somehow exciting, in the manner of an execution.

Their lion was to be devoured by a greater lion.

10.
Demons

I T'S DEMONS, you see," Cassidy said seriously. He was on the floor doing his stretching. Andrea was propped on one elbow on his bed, looking up from her organic chemistry book, suppressing amusement, something she often seemed to do. She pushed a wisp of hair back from her glasses and looked entirely scholarly.

"Do they whisper moral imperatives in your ear?"

"Lovely. I try to explain the dark forces at work within me, and you amuse yourself."

"Oh, I'm sorry, please do go on. And on. And on."

He caught her by an ankle, the good one, and flipped her neatly onto the floor beside him. The back of her neck smelled like a parakeet's tummy, sweet hay and fluff.

"Mmmmm," he said, lost in the pale corn silk of her hair.

She muddled his thought processes, such as they were; he had difficulty studying when she was about. Colors muted and he reached for her without guile or guilt. He adored her and told her so.

She on the other hand had no handle on Quenton Cassidy. He said things occasionally that brought her up short. She would shake her head and say queer duck. He acted not at all like the many boys who had sought her attentions. This one wore a great weariness about the eyes, yet ironically with an incredible well of silly energy bubbling just beneath the surface. He rambled at times, talking in streaks of lucid prose, then lapsed into deep silences from which he could not be retrieved without great effort. He cavorted. He played with her mind.

She had watched him race four times now. He had tried to pass off these competitions as inconsequential, but during those times especially he was lost to her. She wondered where he went, leaving her excluded, lonely, and—could she admit this?—jealous.

She wondered what interior provinces she was not privy to and repeatedly asked him to explain what he was talking about. This she knew: there were times when she drew only polite responses; she could have been for all the world a distant cousin come to visit.

"What do your demons make you do?" she said softly, holding his head and making curls absently with his ragged blond hair. He sighed.

"About sixteen, eighteen miles a day."

"Um." She started to push him away, perturbed at not being taken seriously.

"But sometimes when it is all going good, I mean when it's early May warm and there's cut grass in the air and you've made it through winter okay, not bad sick or anything, then sometimes you can take a deep breath and feel your own heart jumping—*that's right don't look at me like that*—you can feel your own heart in there jumping around like a goddamn bobcat or something; that's when you've just got to get yourself out somewhere and let them loose." Her head cocked at this; she watched him closely.

"Don't try to make me feel funny about this," he said. "You were the one who wanted to know. Besides, you've never been in four-minute shape, not that many people have, so if you think this is all just a crock . . ."

"No," she said quickly. "Go on. I want to hear it."

"They make you want to run through the jungle, baby," he said happily, "cover countryside at a clip, slide by in the night like a scuttling cloud." His eyes had the faraway cast, but his voice quavered in mock solemnity like a Southern tent evangelist. Sensing genuine interest, he picked up the tempo.

"They make you bolt awake in the middle of the night with an involuntary shot of your own true adrenaline, ready to run a hundred miles; we're talking when you're there, now, really there, four-minute shape or better. They make you jittery with the smell of forest, ready to hurdle fallen trees, run down game, leave gore in the bushes . . ."

Her eyes widened.

"And then when you get them all reined in"—he looked at her fiercely—"they make you lay back in the pack, coasting three laps on an old melody . . . and then they make you wail out of the final turn and blow down the last goddamn straightaway like *the midnight train to hell!*"

Although he said it humorously in his mock-religious voice, in his eyes she could see but not quite penetrate limpid ethers of a faraway Elysium, where the otherworldly citizens were without exception vessels of nearly pure spirit: heavyweight prize fighters, rare-air mountain climbers, soon-to-be-martyred saints, and other quiet, sadly ironic purveyors of the Difficult Task.

"You are of course quite mad," she said softly.

"Come," he said, breaking the spell. "We have to meet Mize at the Nineties."

𝒞

"WE ARE SPEAKING of human endeavor and delusional systems," Cassidy said, punctuating with a steady cracking of pistachio nuts. Their second pitcher was almost gone; Thursday-night foosball and pinball background noise nearly precluded conversation altogether.

"Everyone likes to think they have their own little corner; it can be anything: needlepoint, lawn bowling, whatever. Some guy may gratify himself by thinking he's the best goddamn fruit and vegetable manager the A & P ever had. Which is fine. It gives people a sense of worth in a crowded world where everyone feels like part of the scenery. But then mostly they are spared any harrowing glimpses into their own mediocrity. Pillsbury Bake-Off notwithstanding, we'll never really know who makes the best artichoke soufflé in the world, will we?"

"Gotcha. Don't filibuster, tell me Demons," she said.

"Right. The thing is that in track we are painfully and constantly aware of how we stack up, not just with our contemporaries but with our historical counterparts as well. In that regard it's different even from other sports. A basketball player can go out and have a great day and tell himself he's the greatest rebounding forward to ever hit the hardwood, but he'll never really be troubled by the actual truth, will he? Maybe he's just in a weak league. Maybe Jumping Joe Faulks would have eaten him alive thirty years ago. But he'll never know. He'll just have to leave such judgments in the sorry hands of the sportswriters, many of whom it has been pointed out can be bought with a steak." Mizner nodded vigorously from behind a pile of popcorn.

"In track it's all there in black-and-white. Lot of people can't take that kind of pressure; the ego withers in the face of the evidence. We all carry our little credentials around with us; that's why the numbers are so important to us, why we're always talking about them. I am, for instance, four flat point three. The numerals might as well be etched on my forehead. This gentleman here, perhaps you'd like to meet him, is 27:42, also known as 13:21, I believe."

Mizner bowed graciously, half rising. He seemed to be enjoying this immensely.

"A knowledgeable observer might ask yards or meters and it is most assuredly yards," Mizner said. "I'll not puff."

"What?"

"Never mind," Cassidy interrupted. "The point is that we know not only whether we are good, bad, or mediocre, but whether we're first, third, or a hundred and ninety-seventh at any given point. *Track & Field News* tells us whether we want to know or not."

"Assuming we make the lists," Mizner put in.

"That's right. Sometimes it is possible, despite your best efforts and a hundred goddamn miles a week, *not to even exist.*"

"That bothers you, does it?"

"That, my dear, breaks my heart."

"But you can beat almost everyone. We know that, right? Isn't that good? Isn't that what you want?"

"Well, sure. But in my own mind, I know that I'm what a sportswriter would call a 'steady performer.' And it really doesn't matter a whit how many races I win. I haven't even broken four minutes yet. Roger Bannister did that back in 1954. I've spent seven years of my life working hard at this thing and so far I'm . . . average. It happens to others, concert pianists maybe, actors, and the like. But they aren't subject to the cold cruel numbers like we are.

"Let's put it this way," he continued. "There is a fellow right now in New Haven, one in Kansas, one in Boston, one somewhere in Minnesota of all places, and two—Mize is now indicating three—in Oregon who might very reasonably request that I launder their jocks for them. And that's just the United States. There happens to be a young man down in New Zealand right now by the name of John Walton who breathes actual air and eats human food and the son of a bitch has run one mile faster than any human being in the history of the world, 3:49.1 to be exact. I don't believe ol' John'd *let me* wash his jock, do you think, Mize?"

The other runner shook his head solemnly.

"And is there some kind of final point to all this?" Andrea said.

"Depends on what you call a point. It's a simple choice: we can all be good boys and wear our letter sweaters around and get our little degrees and find some nice girl to settle, you know, *down* with . . . take up what a friend of ours calls the hearty challenges of lawn care . . ." Mizner was snickering, but Andrea was solemn. Cassidy stared into his beer.

"Or what? What's your alternative?" She leaned over the table, trying to get him back on track. He looked at her, surprised; his eyes lit up as they had earlier and his voice shook again with excitement.

"Or we can blaze! Become legends in our own time, strike fear in the heart of mediocre talent everywhere! We can scald dogs, put records out of reach! Make the stands gasp as we blow into an unearthly kick from three hundred yards out! We can become God's own messengers delivering the dreaded scrolls! We can race dark Satan till he wheezes fiery cinders down the back straightaway!" He was full into it now.

"They'll speak our names in hushed tones, 'Those guys are animals,' they'll say! We can lay it on the line, bust a gut, show them a clean pair of heels. We can sprint the turn on a spring breeze and feel the winter leave our feet!"

Andrea leaned back in the booth, wide-eyed, and swallowed.

"We can, by God, let our demons loose and *just wail on!*" He threw his head back and let loose a low, eerie cry. Foosball, billiards, and pinballs all stilled suddenly. Mizner, unaware of the sudden quiet, pounded the table in animated agreement.

"Yes, yes, goddamn, that's it! *Wuhail Owwwwnnnn!!*" When he had finished the cry he looked around at the silent blank faces of the various confused fraternity jocks and winced.

"My Lord in heaven," she said, her eyes glistening. But she smiled as she said it, a bemused smile that said perhaps now here was something after all, and even though it was an admission against interest, she had to consider the possibility that there was something here a little . . . out of the ordinary. Later in her life, she would always count that as the moment when she truly fell in love with Quenton Cassidy, a madman vexed and enchanted by ethereal considerations she did not understand, fell in love with him even as he sat, tired from his performance, absently drawing figure eights in the spilled beer.

They were all a tad drunk.

"THAT WAS NICE," Cassidy said. Three days later they were walking back to Doobey Hall in the dark, hand in hand. Though it was November, it was still pleasantly warm out.

"I don't know. It was a little eerie at first. But it was nice to look at the stars," Andrea said.

"People used to do it outside watching the stars all the time until Alexander Graham Bell invented the motel," he said. "But I told you no one would bother us. Very few people know that practice pit is out there. The main one gets a lot of use. I wonder what people used to do back in the old days when the jumpers landed in sawdust."

"Making love in a pole-vault pit." She sighed. "If my mother only knew. She'd be sure to come up with something about 'passion pits' or some such."

"Mothers like those kinds of lines. As if there was guaranteed wisdom in puns and cornpone."

"I suppose."

They walked as slowly as they could without the whole thing

getting silly, both of them having an instinctive sense about preserving good moments. As they neared Doobey Hall, he heard the commotion in back.

"C'mon." He grabbed her hand. "If this is what I think it is, it might be fun."

In the back of the house was a large garage building that had been turned into a recreation and storage area. There was a battered Ping-Pong table, a very old and inoperable jukebox, and some Sidecar Doobey–vintage furniture. Cassidy led Andrea through the door and they stood in the back of the small crowd. A space had been cleared out on the sandy concrete floor to make room for a miniature high-jump arena. Andrea was puzzled.

"What are they . . ." But Cassidy shushed her. Ron "Spider" Gordon was standing at the edge of the open space to their left, his eyes focused on the ridiculous makeshift standards. They had taken two large coatracks and taped coat hangers to hold the horizontal bar, which was an old cane fishing pole. A pile of mattresses made up a comfy-looking landing pit. Cassidy thought of the pole-vault pit, looked down at Andrea with a loud sigh, and was promptly shushed himself. Gordon was going into his routine now, in the manner of all jumpers, clenching and unclenching his fists, mumbling to himself, bending over at the waist and wiggling his hands like gloves with no fingers in them, in general doing the field man's Dance of High Anxiety. Except now it was overtly histrionic, for he was also doing his own voice-over, sotto voce, like a golf-match commentator:

". . . and so, ladies and gentlemen, the pressure is really on the famous Italian high jumper, Ron Don *Giordante,* here in the Olympic finals in this beautiful new stadium in Rome, Italy, in front of thousands of hopeful countrymen . . ."

Andrea did not understand what was going on. The makeshift bar was far over the head of the six-one jumper, and she knew he didn't have enough room to take more than two or three steps.

She got on tiptoes and whispered to Cassidy, who was watching with a big grin on his face.

"Quenton, what's he going to—"

Cassidy shushed her again and nodded at the jumper. "Just watch," he told her.

It was a startling thing to witness, even though most of them had seen it many times. Gordon finished his commentary, leaving off with: "It looks like he's ready . . . yes, there he goes now . . ." The jumper loped in with three casual strides and lifted into the air as if on hidden wings, floating up and over the bar easily, seeming to stay in the air for several seconds before gravity asserted itself. He had cleared the bar by nearly half a foot. Gordon was one of the last to use the western roll, which Cassidy thought far more aesthetically pleasing than the flop, and it was a beautiful thing to watch. Cassidy estimated the bar at 6-5, way over Gordon's head, and though it was nearly a foot below his true capability, seen from up close and in such casual circumstances, it was mildly shocking. The crowd was still applauding good-naturedly as Gordon wallowed around on the mattresses, paralyzed with laughter.

Stoned to the gills, Cassidy thought.

Jim Beale, another jumper, took his place and began going through the antics. Gordon, barely able to control himself, very considerately crawled from the "pit" and began to give the commentary for his colleague. Everyone seemed to be having a wonderful time. Cassidy and Andrea slipped out the back.

"Isn't that something?" he said, shaking his head.

"Weird like everything else around here. I don't think I get it."

"I didn't either, for a while. I've seen the hurdlers, the shot and disc guys doing stuff like that. Never made sense. Then I figured it out. What they're doing is they're *playing* track."

"Playing?"

"Right. See, when you're doing the actual thing itself, it's so competitive and serious, I don't think anybody really has much fun at it. Rarely in practice and *never* in meets. Oh, they like the *idea* of it all right, they like going to competitions, and they like being on a team and the general hullabaloo of being a jock. But when you get right down to it, while you're doing the thing itself, it's not a lot of grins. I can't remember a mile race in my life that was even mildly amusing."

"So what was all that back there about?"

"Well, sometimes Spider or one of the others will be sitting around here and suddenly realize that he *likes* doing what he does. He may have turned it into a compulsion or a job, but it was once something he did as a kid just for the neat sensation it gave him. So Spider will have a few tokes and suddenly realize he *loves* sailing through the air without having to hand someone a boarding pass. I've seen Mobley drink three pitchers and go out and heave his goddamn shot around a playground by moonlight all night. *Weird* stuff like that . . ."

"But they do this every afternoon. I don't see why he would want to go out in some garage . . ."

"It's very simple. Though it looked amazing to us, for him jumping six-five is like strolling around the block. He could do it in his sleep. So, for him to make it into play, all he had to do is drop back several notches off his true capabilities; he puts on a pair of cutoffs, rigs up a stupid cane pole for a bar, and he does . . . *what he does*. It would be like me going out and running a 4:20 mile. I don't know how else to explain it. They do it all the time. Everybody likes to watch, particularly when the high jumpers do it. They make up these fantastic situations, give themselves glamorous foreign names, pretend it's some great vendetta in the Olympics or something . . ."

"But Ron Don *Giordante?*"

"One of the half milers, Benny Vaughn, started that. Everyone on the team now has some foreignized version of his own name. It's a kind of fantasy thing they all get a kick out of."

"Do you have one?"

"Of course. I am Quintus Cassadamius, the famous Greek miler. I'm also somewhat renowned on an imaginary pro bowling tour, but that's another story."

"How about Jerry, does he have a funny name?"

"Sure. Mizerelli, another famous Italian athlete. I was responsible for that one, I guess."

"And how about Bruce Denton?"

"That, my dear, shows how much you know. Bruce Denton is Bruce Denton, the famous American clock cleaner."

A Fan's Notes

THE TREMORS WOKE ANDREA.

She blinked, startled by the unfamiliar surroundings. The tremors continued, rhythmically, far-off, yet deep and powerful, shaking the whole bed. She peered around in the thin yellow dawn light, alarmed but still drowsy, trying to figure out where she was and whether she was in danger. Her hand fell on something warm. It was Quenton Cassidy; she was in his room.

But what was going on? Did they have earthquakes up here in north Florida? She stayed very still, scared, trying to make her sleepy mind work.

Then she figured it out and got really scared.

"Quenton." She shook him gently, urgently. He didn't stir.

"Quenton."

"Hmmmff?"

"Is there something wrong? Baby, wake up, please, Quenton, your heartbeat is shaking the bed . . ."

One bluish-green eye opened and studied her carefully. This was his morning to sleep late. The team would be driving to Jacksonville to catch a plane; the morning run would be just a token.

"Shhh," he murmured softly. "Go back to sleep." She did. The little tremors continued rhythmically; steady liquid drumbeats at precisely thirty-two to the minute.

They did indeed shake the bed.

NOW THAT SOME of the questionable side effects of the lifestyle had actually befallen her, Andrea was far from pleased. For one thing, she wasn't crazy about the idea of staying home on a Saturday night, Mary Tyler Moore or no Mary Tyler Moore.

The team had left at noon and would be gone for days. The USTFF meet was Monday at Penn State, the AAU championships the following Saturday in Chicago. She fretted around her room like a cat on diet pills.

Some of her dateless sorority sisters came by, full of goodwill, not at all unhappy with their plight, and made a pitch for pizza and some tentative prowling around. Andrea demurred as pleasantly as she could.

She was actually pretty miserable, but what really annoyed her was that she didn't know exactly why. She got out a pair of scissors and some old jeans and began to make cut-offs, but tired after one leg and threw the stuff in a corner in a heap. This wasn't like her; not at all. If this was what it was all about, she wanted no part of it.

She cast about her room, distastefully taking in the cute pastel artifacts that had always been her joy. The giant stuffed Snoopy seemed pretty stupid when she thought about it. She felt like giving it a swift kick right in its smiling kisser. Why hadn't she gone with the girls? She knew why. It would have been worse.

Finally she wandered down the hall to the drink machine, came back with a Fresca, sat down at her neat white desk, and took out a legal pad. She had never liked normal girl-type stationery; perhaps because she wrote rambling, philosophical letters rather than bright, quick, newsy ones, and it was embarrassing to stuff twenty or thirty of the little sheets into a small envelope.

In her flowery, nearly illegible handwriting, she wrote:

Dear Alicia,

How are things at horny old Randolph-Macon? If you get this during the middle of the week and don't like to be reminded that the nearest boys are thirty-five miles away, sorry about that.

But don't feel too deprived because here it is Saturday night and little Andrea is sitting in her room at the university voted by Playboy *magazine last year as the number one party school in the country, drinking a Fresca, barely able to hear several nearby live bands and feeling like (excuse the expression) crap.*

And would you like to know where the sports hero is? Okay, but I'm going to tell you anyway because you've probably already figured out this letter is a bitch session. Well, right now he is at the Nittany Lion Inn at Penn State probably trying to charm some Yankee girl with his ridiculous fake Southern accent. Whoever heard of a West Palm Beach drawl? Well, he's got one, but he only trots it out every now and then. He says he got it during summers at his grandparents' in North Carolina. Oh well, he tells me there is really not much fooling around on these trips and why would I have reason to doubt anything said with such sincerity?

He also told me he hated cross-country meets like a plague of boils, but you've never SEEN such a happy traveler packing for a sojourn. Singing, whistling, trying to decide which of those strange little spiked shoes he will take (he has about fifty pairs of them and they all have little stories). Oh yes, he was really upset about leaving, all right.

Leece, what's wrong with me? I've never acted like this before, have I? I wish you were here now. Why did we ever decide to go to different schools?

When he's around I'm not really even conscious of being particularly happy. It just seems kind of normal. But when he has to go off somewhere it's like I cease to do anything but exist until he's back. And it's not like we see each other all that much during the week either. We're both taking a lot of hours this semester and we agreed awhile back that it could really get silly if we let it. So we usually study apart. Still, there's just something about knowing he's not far away.

He says it is going to be worse during the indoor season. He could be gone every weekend if he's running well. And right now he is.

I can't figure it out. It's not that he's beautiful. Sometimes he looks so thin it seems he must be sick or something. And if I say anything, he comes out with these smart-ass comments, like, "It's the lean wolf that leads the pack, baby." Honestly, he can be so condescending I want to just slap him. But then I look in his eyes, and Leece, he's always so tired, so frail looking, it just breaks my heart. Sometimes he catches me looking at him and says, "What?" I say, "Nothing, just thinking."

He says he's "smitten" with me, and I guess he means it. But if there's ever a question of a running thing or an Andrea thing, guess who's second fiddle? Have I ever put up with a boy like this that you can remember?

I wish I could drag him home over Thanksgiving so you could get a look at him, but as usual he's going to be gone. Can't you just see him with Daddy? What if they got into the war or something like that? But I guess they could talk about fishing—Quenton knows all about fish from skin diving in West Palm.

Leece, am I sounding like a little lovesick puppy? Me, the Ice Maiden of Coral Gables High? Brother.

One thing I'll say about him, he didn't flinch when I told him about medical school. Most of the guys I've ever mentioned it to just give me this weak little smile. They're right on the verge of saying something like, oh, you're much too attractive to blah blah blah and if I had a gun right then I would shoot to kill.

I must say Quenton took it right in stride. But then, I guess delusions of grandeur don't startle someone whose real goal in life is to set a world's record (he told me not to EVER EVER tell a soul about that, but telling your twin is not really like telling someone else, is it?).

I don't know, maybe I'm crazy too. I just don't seem to be able to do much of anything about it. Imagine what you'd do if your date wandered around the dance floor at a disco place with a five-dollar bill in his hand telling people he wanted to tip the band but he couldn't find them?

Leece, I was paralyzed. I was the only one, but I couldn't speak, I was laughing so hard. And he didn't care about the weird looks he got, not at all. What is it about this one?

Am I in love, Leece? For true this time, for real?

Love, Andy

12.

The Indictment

IT WAS A DO-NOTHING Thursday afternoon. With a junior college meet coming up the freshmen and sophomores were constrained to playfully jogging five miles. Cassidy and Mizner elected to go the ten-mile course with a few others. The pace would be brisk, around fifty-eight minutes, so extended conversation was necessarily restricted to the first three or four miles. The group headed out on a loop they called "Tobacco Road" because the unpaved road wound through a wooded section south of town replete with shacks, wincing dogs, and barefoot children; it was rumored that the course had been named by Marty Liquori when he was down for the Southeastern Relays. It was like running back in time forty years. But the runners waved to the locals and the locals waved right back. There was a friendliness born of familiarity, and although two entirely different worlds eclipsed each other at that point, by some process of emotional osmosis each had come to respect the other's struggles; there was the homey aroma of country foods in preparation— greens, fritters, and such.

Someone wanted to know what was to be done about Nubbins.

"What about him?" Cassidy asked. "I thought he had become a pillar of the community." They spoke in quick bursts on the exhale.

"Old wine, new bottle," said Hosford, a pale, literary type.

"Haven't you heard the latest?" asked Mizner. "Oh, this is too good. Last Tuesday night, after he won that freshman meet against Auburn, he was feeling pretty full of himself and he goes on a *High Plains Drifter* kick. He dolls himself up in his goddamn Roy Rogers shirt and his shit-kicking boots—"

"I don't see anything so wrong—"

"Wait a minute, let me tell it." Mizner was starting to snicker breathlessly, remembering. "And he had this blanket that he stole from the plane when we went to Atlanta. No lie, this is the honest-to-God truth. He had cut a hole in this piece of Eastern Airlines property to make himself a poncho, see, and then he proceeds to the State Theatre with that birdbrained girlfriend of his, that Betty Sue . . ."

"Aw, come on . . ." Cassidy was not averse to certain brands of extemporaneous craziness.

"Well, trying to be objective, now," Hosford interrupted, "he was making even more of an ass of himself than usual. There was a big crowd in the lobby waiting for the first show to get out. Nubbins kept cavorting around doing his Clint Eastwood material—which is pretty silly considering the little shit is only five eight. Anyway, someone in the crowd would get nervous and giggle, like, you know, from sheer embarrassment. So then Nubbins would get even more loud and rambunctious, thinking he was, you know, *entertaining* them. I mean, I was *there*. I wanted to *hide*, man . . ."

"I think I get the picture," said Cassidy. "Let's pick this pace up a little bit."

THE SHOWER ROOM was a fine place for deep, conspiratorial thinking. Cassidy slumped in the weariness that was his chosen mantle, lost in the hot torrent of water. Mizner, more chipper, sang a gurgling aria at the next nozzle.

"Are you still doing the Honor Court thing?" Cassidy asked from inside his waterfall. His left knee was tormenting him.

"Yeah. Clerk of the Court. That means I get to man the tape recorder and perform other taxing duties. Sure looks good on the résumé, though."

"But you have physical access to the courtroom itself, right? I mean, can you get in whenever you want to, get a hold of letter-head, stuff like that?"

"Sure, that's the job. What's the deal?"

"Oh, just a Classic," he bubbled, "just an all-time classic is what it is . . ."

THE HONOR CODE at Southeastern University followed in that fine old American tradition of overcoming defeat by one, pro-nouncing some unmitigated disaster a resounding triumph, and then, two, smiling pleasantly in the face of even the most crush-ing evidence to the contrary.

Cassidy figured such addlepated stubbornness helped to ex-plain more than a few national lapses like the electoral college, the Eighteenth Amendment, and the current unpleasantness in Indochina. His theory was that it all stemmed from the unrelent-ing and self-damning refusal of the ruling classes to admit that somebody important fucked up. But rest assured, Cassidy would say, that if things get really squirrely—the meltdown *was* a possibility after all, the warhead *could be* armed by accident—some clerk/typist somewhere was definitely going to get the ax.

If such a construct could sustain a silly-assed war in Indochina or a wacko nuclear energy policy, it could surely sustain a student conduct code at a land-grant university in the deep South. The Southeastern University honor code, in brief, commanded far more in the way of belly laughs than respect from the student body.

The program was based upon the presumption that the Honest People were the best sentinels for guarding against Evil and generally preserving the System, whose morality was defined broadly by our Christian Ethics, our American sense of Fair Play, and our sincere conviction that Cheaters Are Only Hurting Themselves. After all, who knew when, some five or so years from now at some important cocktail party, your boss from J. Williston Beckman Widget Company might wander over and request the dimensions of the Parthenon? And then where would you be?

The way it worked was, when you saw someone cribbing, either you were supposed to turn them in or ask them to turn themselves in. There would follow a kind of dollhouse due process in the Student Honor Court, which the law students used to hone their nascent skills.

It was all in good fun, of course. Good fun for everyone except the few unlucky "defendants" who were actually dragged before the child tribunal, slump-shouldered and apparently highly chastened. Generally, the chancellor, exercising his sound discretion, would sentence the malefactor to something like "fifteen makeup credits," thus swelling the rolls of courses like GEO 101 (Rocks for Jocks), MUS 101 (Mozart on a Stick), and other cakewalks. The defendant could then graduate on schedule and go to work in the regional purchasing department of

Wal-Mart, feeling that not only had he paid his debt to society, but also that in a pinch he could identify a feldspar or hum a few bars of *Le Pathétique*.

But just as an aircraft that won't fly is a failure by definition (no matter how comfortable the seats or snazzy the tail design), so Southeastern's honor code was a failure for the simple reason that it inspired more criminality than it prevented.

The wide and airy gulf between ideal and reality was in no instance more clearly demonstrated than the day Cassidy saw an angry student standing hands on hips by an "Honor Fruit Stand," a failed attempt by student government True Believers to sell apples, bananas, and oranges in convenient bins around campus by attaching containers for bright-eyed students to drop their coins into.

The student Cassidy saw that day was upset, glaring at the empty fruit bin (the program had been abandoned quickly for lack of, ah, cash flow), for he turned on his heel and stalked away, exclaiming to no one in particular: "Goddamn! No more free fruit!"

Cassidy was bewildered by the honor system and he generally resented the kind of education he was getting, especially during his first two years at Southeastern, a university large enough to insist on grading humanities examinations by computer.

The way he saw it, mechanical testing per se was not so bad, but the requirements of binary logic coupled with a faculty wholly devoid of imagination led to exam questions that bordered on high comedy. He would never forget one such question. The second quarter of Humanities had concerned itself with the early Greek philosophers, basic religion, architecture, and art (no one ever accused the department of being unambitious). One nearly senile question writer, an associate professor who kept a ferret and was said to be a hoot on a concertina, in a giddy attempt to syllogistically mix his various marbles, offered this poser: *Plato was to Jesus Christ as the Parthenon was to (a) the Appian*

Way; (b) St. Peter's Basilica; (c) the Aqueducts; (d) none of the above.

Cassidy cared little whether he won such contests, left exams in a blind fury, and plotted dark revenge. Time after time he asked instructors about the lunacy of such a system and they were generally sheepish in attempting to defend such vapid academic skullduggery.

Once he was in a section taught by no less than the head of the department. After the midterm exam, Cassidy angrily pointed out the specific page in *Madame Bovary* that demonstrated his answer to a very obscure question was just as correct as the one espoused by the department (and, more important, the computer). The department head, a defeated, gray-headed, and somewhat confused old man, looked up from his unkempt notes and, without the grace of any sort of humor, said between thin white lips:

"No one promised you there would be universal justice, you know."

Cassidy thought: this addled old fart has lost the ability or will to teach, perhaps, but he can still impart useful knowledge. Obliquely; always *obliquely*.

It was late at night and an unmistakable edge of conspiracy tinged the air in Cassidy's room as he unfolded the Plan to Mizner and Hosford. Their jobs would be relatively simple for now; coconspirators were to be recruited and casual gossip was to be chummed around the training table.

But after the scenario was laid out in toto, in spite of Cassidy's frantic efforts to maintain decorum, his room sounded like a cadre of chihuahuas had parachuted into a pigpen.

Nowhere on campus was the honor system more stoutly defended than Farley Hall, the main athletic dorm, where football players in particular professed for it nothing less than True Love, spiritual and enduring. Using the vernacular of the horse track, they discussed at great length the opportunities presented them by such a grab bag of situational ethics. They were cheating their asses off, of course, and doing so with the general high spirits of any playful and energetic group of ne'er-do-wells who discover to their great merriment that someone has wandered off and left the tap unguarded.

The term they used was "riding," which is to say that if one were going to copy from someone else's paper, one would be "riding" that person through the exam. Such a technique was not hard to perfect in the crowded rooms where tests were given. One would, yawning immensely from the strain of all that heavy *pondering*, easily turn one's body this way or that (just trying to loosen up, you understand) and return to one's answer sheet with a string of pure knowledge: 3,2,2,2,1,4,2,4,1. Or was it 2,4,2?

Whether the answers were right or not was entirely dependent on the rider's skill in selecting his "mount." On occasion the mount was a predetermined matter. Generally, though, the selection process was impromptu. A nervous footballer would study the other students carefully as they wandered into the exam room.

"A fat ugly girl is the only horse for me," insisted Harold Sloate, a pig-eyed maniac left guard who eventually made the Atlanta Falcon suicide squad. "Some folks swear by skinny guys with slide rules in they belts, but give me a ugly girl and I'll win the fuggin' Kentucky Derby. One with acne's even better . . ."

The whole process had become more or less a culturally ingrained institution that the athletic department looked upon with a kind of confused admiration (how could the boys, on their own, have come up with this grand way of eliminating expensive tutors?) It reached a point of outright hilarity when some of the more imaginative players showed up at the Farley training table on exam nights with cowboy boots and sterling silver spurs and waited in line for their feed yelling *"Yippeeyi O Kiyaaaay! We gone Riiiide ta-night!"*

Old pig-eyed Sloate topped them all one night by bringing in a forty-five-pound hand-tooled imported brass-horn Western working saddle, complete with fittings and reins. Dragging it up on the coatrack, he ripped off his ten-gallon Stetson and exclaimed to the silently waiting multitudes paused midbite: "Make way, you varmints, there's an EN 201 final tonight and the Pony Express is *comin' through!*" He received a rather nice round of applause, but the next day Dick Doobey called the head dorm counselor and told him in no uncertain terms that although he thought the, um, horsing around was in its own way quite humorous, it was about time to call off the shenanigans. Word was getting around, and some of the more shall we say unathletically inclined faculty members were beginning to make references to measures which, if allowed to gather momentum, just might end up lopping off the head of the proverbial golden goose. In short, it was time to quit pissing in the soup.

Thus it was that the fevered and unexplained local penchant for Western dress that had blossomed so suddenly in Kernsville, died just as suddenly, leaving overstocked haberdashers once more bewildered by the unfathomable vicissitudes of college fashion. The more entrenched trend of jocks "riding" through school, however, remained very much a part of the subculture.

THAT JACK NUBBINS was not getting through exams on his own steam was not in question. In fact he talked about his indiscretions in a booming voice around the training table, mimicking the football players, whom he admired greatly: "Sheeit. I thought he was a thoroughbred, but then I got back muh grade an' it was a measly C! He must have been just a old plow horse, but I swear he had horn-rim glasses an' his own briefcase!" The technique of riding, for all its bravado, was alas only marginally successful. The athletes, using their own limited deductive abilities, figured that the best students were people who *looked* like good students. It never occurred to them that a well-muscled athletic type could pull an A. Neither did they figure that an unattractive female could miss so much as a question or two, what with all the free time she had to devote to her studies. And so it was that the riders were regularly amazed when their nefarious practices netted them mostly Cs, occasional Bs, a few giddy As, and, oh the shock of it all, even some Ds and Es (picture the sad irony of realizing you had superimposed someone else's failure upon your own!). To blunder in such a manner meant not only did you pass up a chance to perhaps guess your way to a better score, but that you couldn't even—hold on to your Stetsons, boys—*cheat right,* for chrissakes!

And if that wasn't enough of a pisser, consider the possibility that one might just be unlucky enough to sit in front of some snit who would take umbrage at one's goggle-eyed yawns and turn one's tender ass in to the exam proctor, which would entail Lord only knows what kind of unpasteurized shit; word had it that the so-called Honor Court even had the power to suspend rubber-necked scholars from school.

It was with considerable trepidation that Jack Nubbins ripped open the envelope whose return address clearly indicated that it issued directly from the Office of the Prosecuting Solicitor of the Southeastern University Honor Court. The letterhead bore not only the standard blindfolded Maiden of Justice, holding her delicate scales, but also somewhat incongruously displayed a smiling caricature of Daryl the Swamp Dawg, the school's unique and unswerving mascot, who seemed to be sniffing at Maid Justice's scales as if tracking down some Alpo.

If the comic impact of the letterhead was lost on Nubbins, the contents were not:

Mr. Jack Nubbins
Room 207, Hiram Doobey Memorial Hall
Kernsville, Florida 32601

Dear Mr. Nubbins:

This office has undertaken an investigation
as a result of certain reports made to this office involving yourself and another student during a recent Physical Science Progress
examination in Humbolt Hall on September 2nd.

Comparison of your paper with the other student in question (whom we now believe innocent
of any wrongdoing) resulted in a Wrong Answer
Correlation (WAC) of 98%. As you perhaps know,
this office makes its decision on whether or not
to prosecute a case based upon the number of
wrong answers two suspects have in common. Generally speaking, a WAC of 60% is considered suf-
ficient to indict.

Your arraignment, therefore, has been set for
the evening of October 12, at 7:30 P.M., in the
Honor Courtroom at the Steven C. Prigman Student
Union. You may be represented by counsel of your
choice or we will appoint a student attorney for
you. Please be prompt.

I feel I should inform you, Mr. Nubbins, that
a 98% WAC is, to my knowledge anyway, a Southeastern University record.

Sincerely yours,
A. William Duva,
Esq.
Solicitor General,
Honor Court

This last gratuitous paragraph was debated extensively, and though he had reservations himself, Cassidy decided to include it, reasoning that by the time Nubbins got to the end of the letter, he would be more or less reduced to a lump of quivering redneck paranoia and therefore quite unlikely to catch such a subtle clue.

Which was the case. Nubbins received the letter on a Friday morning. Cassidy, who had been running a varsity meet in Knoxville, returned Sunday night to find no less than three notes pinned to his door, all from Nubbins. Delighted, he put his bags down and read them right in the hall in the order he figured they arrived:

> *Dear Captin Cassady:*
> *Need to have a pow wow with you when you get back from Tennesee. Please come by my room, which is numbered 207.*
> *—Jack N.*

> *Capt.*
> *Since it is importunt that I speak with you right away, I thought I would say you can come by whether it is late or not (when you get back).*
> *—Jack*

> *Sir:*
> *This is you know who. I have decided to lay low awhile so if you call 392-1458 and ask for Betty Sue Applewhite, she will know where I am because it is still inportunt that I speak with you right away. I have told her what you're voice sounds like so there will be no funny business.*
> *—You Know Who*

On the last note there was a postscript: *P.S. I hope your as good a mouthpiece as everyone says you are.*

$\mathcal{C}$

"Who is it?"

"Cassidy."

"I'm sorry?"

"Cassidy."

Silence. Cassidy sighed, rolled his eyes to the back of his head. "We all live in a yellow submarine," he muttered to the crack in the door.

The door opened slightly wider and he was inspected by tiny frightened eyes.

"Come on, Betty Sue," said Cassidy, brushing by her. Nubbins sat on her bed with a humorous, resigned expression on his face. Cassidy thought: *Too good, Jack. No one would ever think of looking for you in your girlfriend's dorm room.*

"Looks like I've really stepped in it this time, Captain," said Nubbins mournfully. Cassidy sat on the bed beside him and gave him a what's-this-all-about pat on the knee. Betty Sue flicked off *The Dating Game* and perched at the end of the bed with her feet drawn up under her.

Nubbins's ROTC bivouac gear lay in a heap in the corner. Cassidy knew that somewhere in the equipment was Nubbins's cherished purloined issue .45, which he kept loaded at all times. Why he had lugged all the stuff over here, Cassidy couldn't figure. Perhaps Nubbins was thinking along the lines of Ethan Allen and the Green Mountain Boys. Cassidy pictured him set up somewhere in the Ocala National Forest with a regulation latrine, rain gullies, and perimeter warning devices. At night he would forage through the campgrounds, snatching limp hot dogs from vacationing Ohioans.

"Jack," Cassidy said, "you need to get a grip on yourself, son." He put down the letter after a quick pretend read-through. He didn't actually need to read it since he had typed it himself only three days earlier. But Nubbins's fidgeting was keeping him from even doing a good acting job.

"What do you think, Captain? They've got my ass nailed,

don't they?" Nubbins, trying hard to buck up, had adopted a fatalistic outlook. It seemed to comfort him to defer, military style, to Cassidy's very unmilitary captaincy. This dorm room was his last stand before the bastards stormed the walls; his own personal Alamo. He envisioned perhaps a ballad about himself.

"Well, Jack, I'll lay it on the line to ya. It does *look* pretty bad." Nubbins lowered his head and nodded.

"But I'll tell ya somethin' else," Cassidy continued, his voice quavering with emotion, "I've gotten some sons a bitches out of jams a helluva lot worse than this!" He gestured at the letter with the disdain of a man who saw paper threats for what they were, a man who dealt with his own crystalline brand of reality, using insight gained only where such knowledge is available: through hours in the breech, days on the firing line, weeks behind the eight ball. What's more, he was clearly a man who did not abandon his friends when, as the attorney general himself used to say (before *his* indictment), the going got tough.

"You no doubt have heard about my work on the defense side in the Honor Court?" Cassidy asked with a trace of pride. Nubbins became suddenly animated.

"Why, they say that you're—"

Cassidy held up a hand; he was not a man who needed idle flattery.

"But you'll take my case?" Nubbins asked, wide-eyed.

"Goddamn right I will!" Cassidy stuck his jaw out.

Nubbins peered up at his counsel with relief and gratitude, brushed manfully at his glistening eyes, and tried to clear his throat.

"And you think we can win?" he croaked.

"Does a pigeon walk funny?"

13

The Trial

B UOYED BY HIS ATTORNEY'S CONFIDENCE, Nubbins returned
warily to Doobey Hall. After all, hadn't he been hearing for
weeks tales of Cassidy's remarkable courtroom prowess? Still, in
those long hours between their numerous conferences, Nubbins's
spirits faltered. He was in considerable and very real distress
most of the time.

His thinking went like this: if worst came to worst and he
found himself suspended from the university, it would cost him a
year redshirting somewhere else, assuming that another school
would take a convicted academic scoundrel. But he knew that
even if he were able to transfer, he would have lost a great deal
by not graduating from Southeastern (Coach Cornwall had gone
out on a limb just to get him admitted on academic probation).

And there was the additional shame of facing the many members of the Nubbins tribe, all of whom were as proud as they were baffled that some fancy-Dan university would not only let one of their wretched clan in, but would actually pay him real money just for pursuing an activity many of them had cultivated involuntarily while eluding various game officials, marine patrolmen, and deputy sheriffs; namely, hightailing it on foot. That this brilliant progeny should be shipped home in disgrace for some academic indiscretion would, of course, be accepted with a degree of sympathy and fatalism (it *had* been too good to be true after all), but on the other hand there would be a lingering suspicion that somehow the scatterbrained young'un had blown his big chance to become president.

Such was the young runner's discomfiture that Cassidy considered calling the whole thing off. An All-time Classic in the making was one thing, but watching this central Florida palmetto tramper sitting mute and bug-eyed over his scrambled eggs every morning was a bit more than Cassidy really needed in the way of humorous feedback. The kid was hooked, living out this awful fantasy in isolation while the others looked on with growing alarm. They all just wanted to bring the scenario to its dramatic conclusion, have a good laugh, and then let the poor boob down (hoping to God he was unarmed at the Moment of Truth). But having set the trial date themselves, they were stuck with it. Cassidy told Nubbins cockily that he had filed a motion to move the case along quickly and that on the night in question they would "wrap this turkey up once and for all."

For two more days Nubbins sweated out his future. The more frantic he became, the more unsure the plotters became. Mizner brought up the unpleasant thought that Jack might become so depressed he would decide to chew on the end of his own .45. Who would want to live with that?

Cassidy had no doubts who would be damned if that happened. But he knew Nubbins well. Cassidy figured anyone who would squat with his ass in freezing water for three hours before dawn just for the chance to blast the feathers off a hapless mallard could damn well keep a date with Maid Justice without cracking. Cassidy kept everyone as calm as he could.

But finally even Hosford, the most vindictive of the puppeteers, caught a case of nerves.

"Geez, do you think we maybe ought to tell him? He's getting a little flaky around the edges."

"I think he'll make it okay," said Cassidy, trying to memorize his lines. "He's only got until tomorrow night."

"Yeah, but let me tell you. He came up to me this morning and started talking real strange. In this real cocky way—you know how he is—he starts telling me what a great lawyer you are and how he had personally seen you get people off who were guiltier than hell . . ." He looked at Cassidy. "You've never tried any cases for real, have you?"

"Never been in a courtroom," Cassidy chirped, studying his script.

"Anyway, he told me you had pull with the chancellor, and that you and this Duva guy, the prosecutor, drink beer together all the . . ."

"Who is a figment, of course."

"A figment?"

"Of my own fevered imagination."

"Yes, well, he's doing everything but hyperventilating. You really think he'll do all right?"

"I think he'll make an excellent defendant. However, I have grave doubts—"

"Doubts?"

"About counsel's ability to bring home the bacon."

THEY WERE ALL THERE. Mizner wearing his official blazer with the court seal over the pocket, Cassidy in an attorneyish double-breaster, the chancellor in his black robes and stern wire-rims, the prosecutor in a rather obnoxiously dashing sports jacket, and Betty Sue Whatsherface, whom Nubbins had timidly asked be allowed to sit in on the "proceedings." And then there was Nubbins himself. Cassidy had told him to dress conservatively, using his own judgment. The lad wore a plain white shirt and black knit tie, and for his jacket selected a smart suede cowboy job with rather short fringe on the sleeves. The effect was prairie/formal: Daniel Boone addressing a joint session of Congress. The various participants had been carefully screened by Cassidy and Mizner. There were a few others in the room who had simply heard about the spoof—despite the harsh oath of secrecy—and had begged to watch. All in all, the courtroom, which was never used for real trials at night, was about half full.

The chancellor was a contradiction in terms: a law student with a sense of humor. He generously offered to lend his solemn presence to the occasion in exchange for a print of the eight-by-ten glossy Cassidy was having taken of the defendant and the various court officials. For this purpose a friend of Mizner's was introduced to Nubbins as the "court photographer" who was going to "photograph key points in the proceedings for the record." Nubbins nodded with the bland assent of a three-time loser being fingerprinted.

Selecting the prosecutor had been difficult. Surprisingly, several sadistic individuals had clamored for the job. There resulted some hilarious tryouts during which Cassidy found himself doing a reasonably bitchy director: "Look, baby, you've got to give me some *hostility*, for chrissakes. This guy is a lousy cheater and you're a self-righteous asshole, so let's emote that to me, baby, eee-mote. Okay, let's take if from if this treachery goes unscathed, our very foundations of self-government et cetera et cetera . . ."

Eventually everyone got into the act. The rejects for the prosecutor's job got to be the bailiff and the stenographer. Everyone dressed for his part with uncanny professionalism. It looked like *Divorce Court* without commercials.

Cassidy thought the room itself was the perfect backdrop. In the manner of all effective courtrooms (as well as legislative chambers and religious edifices) it was designed to impress upon the single blinking supplicant that there was a *power* out there, a force all around that was fierce and swift and terrible in its retribution, an ascendancy that would—should he so much as fart without permission—crush him like the vermin he knew in his heart he was.

How polished mahogany could have such a debilitating effect upon the individual spirit, Cassidy could not figure, but that it did there was no doubt, for here beside him sat this quaking leather-fringed buffoon, sweating like a field hand and looking for all the world like he would leap straight up and grab on to a light fixture if someone so much as said "boo." In fact, when the chancellor's gavel went down with a *thwack* Nubbins popped up like overdue toast. Cassidy reached over with a reassuring lawyerly hand.

"All right, next matter. What is this case?" said the chancellor.

"Case number 72-3689, Your Honor. Student Body versus Jack Nubbins. Three witnesses. WAC of ninety-eight percent."

The judge looked up from the papers he was studying and made a low whistle, obviously impressed.

"Ninety-eight percent, why, that would be a . . ."

"That's right, Your Honor, a . . ."

". . . record, wouldn't it?"

"Record, yes, sir. We checked."

They brought if off with such pristine sincerity, these volunteer thespians, that Cassidy swelled with pride. He had written all the lines himself for this far-Off-Broadway production and his people were doing him proud. They all (except Cassidy) had scripts in front of them in legal folders, but no one seemed to need them.

The script at this point called for the judge to request the prosecutor to approach the bench. This gave Cassidy a chance to lean over and inform Nubbins that this judge was not the one he usually dealt with. There was mention of illness. They would have to feel their way along but not to worry because—

"Mr. Cassidy," the chancellor was interrupting. "I think it only fair to inform you that I will not allow you to get away with the kind of monkeyshines that I understand are your very trademark."

"Judge, I'm just a simple country lawyer and I'm sure that the Court knows I would never stoop to—"

"You know precisely what I mean. Just watch it!"

"Yes, sir!" Cassidy leaned over and whispered to Nubbins: "I was afraid of something like this."

As the hearing went on, Cassidy did not look at any of his confederates around the room. If their eyes locked for more than a split second, great uncontrollable quakes would start deep in his diaphragm and, if unchecked, very quickly the whole mad, delicately balanced façade would crumble in premature hilarity. To cover himself, a few times he feigned coughing spells. He needn't have gone to the trouble, actually, for Nubbins, sensing things were not going well for the home team, was staring straight ahead in a melancholy trance. He now knew his lawyer, brilliant though he might be, was out of favor with this particular judge. Even as Cassidy rose to voice his objections, he was being overruled. And Nubbins could not remember having stumbled upon a human being, a total stranger at that, who obviously felt such open and hostile loathing for him as the natty prosecutor. It was hard to imagine that the fellow did not have some grave mental problem, such was his rancor. It seemed as though he might at any moment leap across counsel table and come at Nubbins with a hidden dagger. But apparently this cruel and clever antagonist had no need for such weapons; his objections were universally taken under consideration and just as universally sustained by the smiling judge. With each such telling point the prosecutor would look over, resplendent in his ensemble, and openly sneer at Nubbins and his obviously overrated attorney. Nubbins was going deeper and deeper into a kind of shock. He had never been in a situation where the cards had been so obviously, so inexorably, so uniformly stacked against him. His attorney, he now realized, was fighting a holding action against implacable odds; he was simply outmanned by the same immutable stars that had brought Nubbins into this courtroom in the first place.

Everyone was due for an unmitigated shitstorm at some time in his life, Nubbins figured, and this was clearly his turn.

Attorney Cassidy, struggling valiantly in this lost cause, was making motions that the entranced Nubbins could not have possibly paid any attention to, else he would have detected the faint but unmistakable aroma of rotten halibut on the breeze.

"Your Honor, I would like to make a motion e pluribus unum—"

"I object! He can't move for e pluribus unum in this proceeding. There isn't even a jury empaneled!"

"Sustained."

"Well then, Judge, I would like to request a quid pro quo in order to—"

"Objection! Clearly improper before the defendant takes the stand."

"Sustained. Mr. Cassidy, I must warn you, sir! Please sit down!"

This went on long enough for Nubbins to clearly get the drift. Then Cassidy requested a recess in order to discuss something important with his client. Even this request was only grudgingly granted. As a group, all the court personnel, the spectators, and even Nubbins's timid girlfriend (sensing somehow that it was the thing to do) rumbled out of the room leaving lawyer and client alone in the large chamber. Cassidy, his borrowed horn-rims cocked up on his forehead, rubbed his weary lawyer eyes.

"Well, Jack, I guess you can see things aren't going so hot."

"Yeah, that judge doesn't like you one *little* bit. And the prosecuting one! What's he got against me anyway? I don't know him from Adam's nephew."

"Just doing his job, Jack, doing his job. But the chancellor. I think we may have a chance with him. He seems perturbed that we're dragging this thing out with a full-blown trial. Another lawyer told me once he likes to see people come in and lay it on the line. Otherwise, if you go through a trial and he still finds you guilty, he really throws the book at you."

"What do you think we ought to do?"

"I'm thinking we ought to go ahead and plead guilty and throw ourselves on the mercy of the court." *Steady*, he thought. *Burst out laughing now and you'll blow the whole thing.*

"Well, you're the boss, you know that. We've come this far . . ."

"Listen, Jack, I want you to know—"

"Hey, I know. Listen, I thought you were doing a great job. Some of those motions, man . . ."

"Yeah. I should have won a couple of them at least. Anyway, let's give it a go. And Jack . . ."

"Yeah?"

"Remember, no matter what happens, I was there when you needed me." They shook hands solemnly. Nubbins was still sure he had a fine lawyer. Cassidy notified the bailiff and everyone was called back in. Defense counsel advised the Court that his client wished to change his plea to guilty as charged, and to ask for the mercy of the Court. He could barely get the words out. He dared not look at anyone as he spoke; they were all holding it together with sheer willpower.

The judge seemed relieved by this announcement and thanked Cassidy for sparing the Court a "long and arduous trial." He then thanked the court personnel for their hard work. He requested that Nubbins rise with his attorney while he pronounced sentence.

Since Cassidy had put several hours of work into the sentencing speech, he was gratified to see it delivered with the loving attention of a fine performer.

"Mr. Nubbins," the chancellor began, removing his spectacles, "I must admit that I have often wondered why we so seldom see athletes in here, what with all the speculation that goes on about the ethics of those who reside in Farley Hall. I know I should not let my personal feelings become involved, but I've always sensed that you jocks think you run this institution. Now, I'm not a varsity athlete myself, Mr. Nubbins—oh, in high school I played a little basketball and was conference champion in the two hundred butterfly, but I guess when they got around to handing out the scholarships . . . Oh well, that's neither here nor there. What I'm here to tell you this evening, Mr. Nubbins, is that I am now a serious student here at Southeastern, and there are many of us serious students here, Mr. Nubbins, students who don't get their way paid by rich uncle over in Farley Hall, read me? It's too bad that you have to bear the brunt for all the ones who have done the same thing you have and gotten away with it, but I don't know any other way to bring the message home that *you jocks don't run this campus!*"

He paused, as if regaining his composure somewhat, and added as an almost understood afterthought: "We politicos do."

"This is your sentence, Mr. Nubbins: you are hereby suspended from this university indefinitely."

There was a perfect silence in the courtroom.

Such was the demented sincerity of this last diatribe that many of the onwatchers, though they knew it was a farce, were actually a little mortified at the chancellor's rancor. There was much sullen gaping going on, as if no one knew exactly how to end the whole ordeal. Nubbins just stood quaking, his mouth a small, dark cave. He stared unbelieving at the still-bristling judge.

Suddenly the "court photographer" ran out of the spectator's section, snapped a flash picture of Cassidy and Nubbins, and scurried back. Cassidy could no longer control himself. Weakly, he bent at the waist, held his stomach with both hands, and began making deep, resonant yelps not unlike the fierce mating call of the male peacock. Nubbins looked over at him; his own lawyer found the penalty so harsh he could not keep from laughing!

That broke the dam, of course, and the entire courtroom was quickly engulfed in a giant spasm of raucous laughter. With a wild clamor, the teary-eyed actors and half-paralyzed spectators began stumbling over feebly to shake hands with the defendant and pound his back gleefully.

The little runner's wide eyes did not blink as his head swiveled back and forth, a berserk lighthouse. He thought, *How can anyone be so cruel as to actually enjoy seeing me get booted out of school? And my own lawyer is still laughing; did he find it amusing too?*

Even the judge, black robes flowing, came down and threw his arm around Nubbins's shoulders, barking all the while.

Betty Sue sat amid the considerable confusion with a vague smile on her face, wondering what in the bejesus was going on. She knew one thing: old Jack had done something wonderful and she was very proud.

14.

Indoors

WINTER ARRIVED in the Panhandle in its usual desultory fashion; a time of bright, cool days, chilly rains, fading landscapes. The harsh glare of those cloudless days muted the grass, the moss-draped oaks, and sometimes the higher callings of the spirit.

"It is easier to train hard up North," Denton told them. "Snow is snow. You either run in it or you don't. It gives you something to go against, an irritant. But also a stimulus, if you know what I mean. Down here the freezing rain runs down your neck one day, next day you'd think spring had sprung in January."

"What's wrong with that?" Cassidy asked.

"Such a winter is always getting your hopes up."

But winter was the indoor season and for Cassidy it was a

time of renewed hopes. He had had his cross-country drubbings; now he longed to turkey-trot a victory lap.

"I've just had an odd thought," said Cassidy, looking out the oval porthole, enjoying the crisp, heady vacuum of jet flight.

"Do tell." Denton looked up from his botany journal.

"Here we are flying several miles high across the Eastern seaboard—look, that must be Savannah—flying across the Eastern seaboard a couple of thousand miles at a cost of several hundreds of dollars so that we can take off our street clothes, put on little kangaroo-skin slippers that weigh about three ounces each, and shag ass around a little board track for exactly one mile—two in your case. And there are these people, thousands of them, who live in skyscrapers of block and glass, and who will pay money to come and watch us do it. This is the culmination of man's technology, zipping us along at six hundred miles per hour . . ."

"Maybe it just means that civilization has progressed to the point where it can afford even the most esoteric of specialties, even in sports. We are the athletic equivalent of pickled bees knees in the gourmet section at the Winn Dixie."

"Hah." This last took Cassidy by surprise. He looked over and Denton smiled back sweetly, letting Cassidy know once more that there are some people you do not take for granted, even for a second.

Cross-country had ended surprisingly. At the AAU National Championships in Chicago's Washington Park, Cassidy, to his own great surprise, kept the leaders in view almost the entire race, finishing with frozen slush halfway up his calves in fifteenth place, four ahead of Mizner. He had never beaten the younger runner at any distance over two miles. Denton won the race with such ease that the other top cross-country men, stacked up in the finish chute, simply shook their heads in discouragement even as they bent to their knees still gasping from the effort. Denton seemed more delighted with Cassidy's finish than he was to win yet another national title. He even did a little jig as Cassidy, sprinting through the mud to edge out an Oregon runner, sailed into the chute with a grimace. A few seconds later they were all standing around in the slush, laughing though still out of breath, kicking mud at one another. Even Mizner, disappointed as he was, seemed to have a good time, though Cassidy could see he was worried.

Cross-country, to Cassidy's immense relief, was over for another year.

"IN LANE SIX, wearing number 278, from Southern California, the PAC champion . . ."

The announcer was going into the introduction for the two-mile, the longest running event in the Millrose Games in Madison Square Garden. Cassidy jogged out onto the track to take Denton's sweats from him. The other two-milers milled around with constrained nervousness; some trotted back and forth in their lanes, some bounced up and down. It was a time of cruel stress. One race represented months of training; each step the product of many miles of preparation. They would have thought of this race countless times, some of them running it in bits and pieces during interval training or overdistance. They would have thought of creeping up to Denton's shoulder with a lap to go; that sort of fantasy could get them through long hours on the roads at night. But with the starting gun only seconds away, their heads were roaring with anticipation and anguish. They wanted to be into it. They wanted to be over it. The race itself was bearable, for that they had trained. The waiting, however, was hell on square wheels. Denton handed Cassidy the navy blue sweat top with USA in red and white piping, a status symbol, the sign of a member of a national team. Two other runners in the field wore the same kind of sweats; this would not be a stroll.

"Hang in there," Cassidy said quietly.

"Yeah." Denton was glazed over in concentration, even for a

race that he surely couldn't consider very important. He was not a classical indoor runner; both he and Cassidy were too tall to maneuver the banked turns as easily as the shorter runners. And Denton never, never took a race for granted. Though he said little, Cassidy knew he was appreciative of having someone there to offer small comforts.

"In lane three, two-time AAU six-mile champion, one-time three-mile champion, twice a member of our Olympic team . . ."

They were getting into the heavies now. Cassidy took the sweats, swatted Denton on the rear, and jogged to the infield to watch.

"And in lane one . . ."

The crowd was already beginning to rumble.

". . . representing Southeastern University Track Club and the United States . . ." It was difficult to hear now. *". . . ladies and gentlemen, the Olympic gold medalist in the five-thousand-meter run . . ."* Bruce Denton trotted forward in his lane with a serene little wave even though he had not heard his name. No one had. This was what that one perfectly executed race and the thousands of miles of training it required had earned him: the right to have his name lost in the uncontrolled frenzy of this crowd. Denton was thinking: *I only won by three yards.*

Such adulation had roared down for him many times since he first heard it sprinting down the straightaway in the Olympic stadium. He would surely hear it many times again in his life. But as Denton trotted out and wistfully accepted it once more, Quenton Cassidy thought his smile seemed sad indeed.

". . . and entering the final lap now, ladies and gentlemen . . ." The starter's gun went off with a loud crack: gun lap. *". . . Gold medalist Bruce Denton followed by . . ."* It was all meaningless. The pack was a full half-lap behind, running for places. Denton cavorted. He ran wide up on the banked turn and zipped back down onto

the straightaway, playing roller coaster. Cassidy shook his head. Here he was racing some of the best distance men in the country, and he was playing around.

When Denton crossed the finish line, Cassidy trotted up alongside and handed him the sweats. Denton, despite the ease with which be had won, was in no condition to talk; he took the sweats, grinned at Cassidy, and jogged on. He occasionally waved as a section of the audience stood to cheer when he passed beneath them. Cassidy shook his head, ran slowly to the outer hallway to complete his warm-up; his race was in thirty-five minutes, according to the almost universally unreliable schedule.

Cassidy had ripped the order of events out of the program and was careful to check his watch often. By listening to the announcer, he would be able to tell how far behind the meet was running and thus time his warm-up accurately. The large cold hallway did not make a complete circuit, but it was roomy; brightly colored sweat suits flashed by at various speeds. Cassidy had jogged the elliptical half-circle three times by the time Denton came out to find him. Even now his face was red, his voice hoarse from the harsh smoky air.

"Want company?" It was a rhetorical question. Here in this chilly, foreign environment, with so many talented athletes everywhere, it was easy to get psyched out. Cassidy knew no one here except Bruce. He was already beginning to ask himself the eternal self-doubt question: What Am I Doing Here? But now he wasn't just some nobody in a Southeastern University sweat suit jogging back and forth, he was "the guy with Bruce Denton." His stride took on a proud bounce.

"Do you know any of these guys in the mile?" he asked Denton. The older runner took the list and studied it as they ran.

"Well, Marcel Philippe you know. He's a Fordham guy, can't be in real good shape yet. O'Rork I'm sure you remember; Kerry Ellison, Texas El Paso: tough cookie. Those guys get in shape early like we do. I'd say he's the man to watch."

"I didn't think he—"

"He doesn't run on the cross-country team, is why you didn't see him at nationals. They have a bunch of true six-milers, so he doesn't have to. No, he'll be in shape. Wouldn't be here otherwise."

"Yeah, but what about old—"

"Liquori is scratched."

"Scratched? Jeez . . ."

"Breaks your heart, doesn't it? I talked to him a few minutes ago. He is in pretty good shape but he sprained his ankle a few days ago. I hate to say this, but it looks like you might have a chance to take all the marbles."

"Bruce, I . . ." His forehead wrinkled with concern. "Bruce, the Wanamaker Mile . . ."

"Look. This is the way it happens. You keep at it hard, just like you've been doing. You hang around the fringes waiting for your chance. When it comes you go for it, hard. You do good, that gets you psyched. You go back, work even harder . . ." He stopped for a moment, reflected, then laughed. "Hell, I don't know. Who the hell knows?"

"The Millrose mile . . ."

"All I know is that you could win the thing. Your best races are the ones where you just relax and let it flow. You've got great speed, Cass. Jeez, I wish I had it. All you have to do is keep from fretting it away early. It doesn't do any good anyway, indoors especially. Avoid hassles; when you make a move, go around the problems and stay around them. You can run behind just fine so long as you don't get lulled into a bad place late in the race. If you're in a good spot, don't panic even if you're a little crowded. Hang in there and hum a little tune, talk to yourself, look at the girls, *anything* . . . just stay in contact and get yourself to a good position with two laps to go. Don't wait until it's too late to get to your spot. You just don't make up really big gaps indoors, especially on this track."

"Yeah, it's a little slow, isn't it?"

"It's pretty bad for the sprinters, but okay for us. A little spongy is all. I don't think it will affect you that much, but since you push off strongly from your calves you might try to get a little more float out of your stride, instead of trying to get oomph from the track. It doesn't have it to give."

"Got it. Want to do some striders with me?"

"Striders? Striders? Hell, I just did an 8:32 deuce and you want me to do striders with you just to keep you company?" He took off down the concrete hallway in a sprint, scattering runners in all directions. Cassidy smiled; it was always a great feeling to have it over with.

"*. . . FOUR LAPS TO GO and it's O'Rork of East Tennessee, Philippe of Fordham, Ellison, Cassidy, Wheeler, and Hector Ortiz of Western Kentucky . . .*"

Cassidy tried to make his mind work. Eleven laps to the mile, two and three quarters equals one regular lap. Unaccustomed to gauging fatigue versus distance remaining on an indoor track, he had to make conversions as he went along. A runner is a miser, spending the pennies of his energy with great stinginess, constantly wanting to know how much he has spent and how much longer he will be expected to pay. He wants to be broke at precisely the moment he no longer needs his coin.

He calculated: outdoors it would be the third lap. For the time being he was content to tuck in with the middle of the pack and wait for something to happen. The pace had not been impressive; Cassidy felt comfortable with it. They had gone through the half in 2:02 in a bunch. Each time he went by the far turn, Bruce Denton, archfan, was one voice among fifteen thousand who called just for him. Denton yelled things that were not in the least irritating like most of the things you hear during a race (things like "pick it up, pick it up" or "faster,

faster, don't let them get away"), things that make the runner think: *If you think it's so damn slow, why don't you goddamn well get out here and "pick it up" yourself.*

Instead, Denton said: "Good pace, Cass, hang right there!" Or: "Good position, stay alert . . ." To the runner, traveling at a dizzying fifteen miles per hour around a tiny oval track, entranced by pace concentration, the idea of staying alert seemed positively brilliant.

With no warning and but two laps to go, Kerry Ellison surged powerfully. His brown legs flashed smoothly as he let out a burst of brutal speed. Cassidy responded immediately by pulling out, but he had to wait for a straightaway to pass the two runners in front of him. Damn! Then he realized with a sinking heart what Denton had said to him on each of the last two laps: "Move up now. Move up now."

But he had not heeded. Now he was just where he didn't want to be, in a bad position late in the race.

The gun went off as they banked into the penultimate turn. By now Cassidy had pulled back to within ten yards of the flying Texan. With growing confidence he crept steadily up to Ellison's shoulder, using the entire far straight to do it, but feeling—though fatigued from the pace—that he had spirit left. He had gotten out of the jam by responding immediately to Ellison's bid and he seemed to have something left to throw into it. He was excited and just as curious as the spectators to find out what was going to happen. The crowd, on its feet since the crack of the gun, didn't seem to care who won. They just wanted a race.

The excitement of the approaching finish yarn, as always, caused a little prickly feeling at the back of his neck. Cassidy started to pass on the final turn, but just as he pulled up and began the effort, he heard Denton through the din: "NO!" That was all he said. This time Cassidy heard.

He hung on Ellison's shoulder all through the tiny turn and

with a gasp flung himself out and into the final straight. Ellison was not finished either; he pumped smoothly and leaned into his final sprint. But Quenton Cassidy was by far the faster kicker. He easily gained seven yards on Ellison in the last straight. From the crowd came a subdued roar that signified the anticlimax. Denton jumped up onto the track and trotted up to where Cassidy was bent over in the familiar gasping position.

"Don't grab those knees, boy," he shouted above the din. "Here are your sweats, get 'em on. But don't you grab those knees, though, because you got to run a little of that off. You have just become the Wanamaker Mile champion and you got to let them *know* . . ."

Cassidy's face was the old fire-engine color and his breathing still desperate.

"Know. What?" He tried to jog, but it felt as if his spine were made of bamboo. Nothing worked properly, lactic acid bound him into a solid block. He could not swing his arms.

"That it feels GOOOOD!" Denton seemed much happier at the moment than his young friend.

ON THE PLANE, Cassidy was a zombie again, smiling vacantly but apparently unable to assimilate what was going on around him. They had gone out to eat and hadn't gotten to bed until two in the morning. Denton insisted they take a token morning run, so they clomped around stiffly in the gray Manhattan morning. Denton assured him most muggers did not work early.

Cassidy barely made it to his seat. The stewardess woke him to ask if he wanted breakfast—he did—and woke him again a few minutes later when she brought it. When they arrived in Philadelphia, Denton woke him again.

"Hey, champ, end of the line. All milers off." Cassidy mumbled something and then snoozed while the other passengers slowly departed. He nodded off gently while Denton got a cab

and then slept soundly all the way to the hotel as Denton sat in
the front seat and chatted with the driver.

"Whatz wrong wid yer buddy?" the driver asked.

"Wanamaker's Syndrome," Denton said. "Subclinical. Real
pity is, the guy used to be a fine athlete."

"Too bad," clucked the driver.

"HEY, RIP! Time for grub. Let's get it on." It was Denton again.

Cassidy thought: *He's enjoying himself, there's no doubt about it.*

"I don't think I'm going to live," he told Denton.

"They've got great clam chowder at this place only a couple
of blocks away," said Denton, as he dressed. "Also a nice little rib-
eye steak that I, for one, would not miss on a bet."

"What the hell is that?" Cassidy pointed out the window.

"That, my boy, is snow. White stuff that falls from God. It
won't hurt you actually, as long as you don't swallow any or carry
it in your pocket. Some people claim it has magical powers. Try
to put on long wooden planks and slide on it. Personally I don't
think it will catch on. Come *on*! Get your ass in gear, I'm starving."

Despite himself, once they were out in the cold air walking to
the restaurant Cassidy started to feel better. After he had some
tea, he tried to snap out of it altogether.

"I don't understand how I can have jet lag in my own time
zone. How do you do this all winter?"

"This?" Denton crumbled some crackers into his chowder.
"This, my boy, is fine. This is your reward for getting into good
shape early, because these Northern sharpies won't fly you in
from the coast or Florida to run in their shows unless they know
you can produce. Hell, they could get a fairly respectable field in
the mile or deuce from the New York–Boston area if they had to.
We furnish an element of the exotic. You'd best get used to the
idea if you keep winning. A 4:01.3 is not a bad time, indoors.

Especially on that sponge-cake track in the Garden. That might be worth, oh—"

"Come on, Bruce . . ."

"That might be worth a three—"

"Cut it out, Bruce!"

"A 3:58 or so, Cass." He looked up seriously from his chowder.

Cassidy sipped his tea morosely. These things were not to be bantered about lightly. It was bad luck to put your mouth on times your feet couldn't reach. Denton got up to talk to someone at the cashier.

"Who was that?" Cassidy asked.

"Someone who is going to make your evening interesting."

"Come on . . ."

"Just don't try any of that last straightaway kicking crap like last night or you'll hear someone behind you snickering."

"Bruce, who . . ."

"Sammy Bair."

"Shit."

THE PHILADELPHIA MEET was a classic second-meet-of-the-weekend letdown. Denton won in 8:44 from an undistinguished field and Cassidy ran 4:05.2 for second. Sam Bair didn't laugh at him but he might as well have.

By the time they were seated on the plane the next morning, Cassidy was back in his walking coma.

"You gonna have breakfast?" chirped Denton as they strapped in. "I mean if you don't want her to wake you . . ."

"Bruce, you can have my goddamn breakfast. Why don't you just try to cheer up a little?" He dropped off into a sleep that didn't abate until they reached Atlanta, where they changed planes.

He didn't dream.

15.
Casualty

THE SPLENETIC FIREPLUG OF A NURSE turned the page of her *Cosmo* juicily, saw it was going to get pretty good, and elected to take a pit stop before going on. The article was entitled: "Your S[exual] Q[uotient]: Rating Yourself in the Boudoir."

As soon as she toddled off, the vigilant Quenton Cassidy tossed aside his *National Geographic* ("I Lived With the Bagharack Mountain Apes" by Dr. Jane Tully-Wells, one for the neo-Freudians, he thought), grabbed the aromatic flat box, and sprinted for the stairwell. This was past visiting hours. This was illegal. This was keeno neato fun.

He sashayed into Mizner's room with the box on his upturned fingers, singing in a lusty though muted voice: "Cara mia whaaay . . ."

Mizner: "Shhhh!"

Cassidy moaned: "There's a village called Surrentohhh . . ."

Mizner: "That goddamn old bat of a—"

"In the can."

"Oh."

Mizner sat up in bed, pale in his old sweatshirt, a faded dusty purple job with the traditional winged foot and the nearly illegible legend: POMPANO BEACH TRACK. Cassidy scurried around setting up. He stuffed a towel in the crack under the door. He pulled up a chair and produced with considerable flourish the two cans of beer, one from each pocket. Mizner applauded quietly. Had Cassidy stood still for just a moment and really looked at his friend, real tears might have slid down his fleshless cheekbones. Mizner was what they called a "Hurtin' Swamp Dawg." But he told Cassidy: "You brang sich joy into mah hort." In a dreamy, nearly dopey voice this was.

They attacked the disk, which—although containing mostly squashed tomatoes and fermented animal parts—the Italians will scarcely claim. Even after Mizner threw in his napkin, Cassidy kept on eating, primarily because he wanted something to do. He was still unstable here.

"So tell me about Millrose, dammit. Every detail. Do not stint. Do not leave out a spike hole or a careless elbow," Mizner said impatiently.

"The *Kernsville Sun* captured it quite well actually," Cassidy said, "following their normal tradition of printing straight wire copy, despite the fact two local heroes did good. Let's see, Liquori scratched, bless his little heart. No furriners, for some reason— maybe immigration rounded 'em all up or something—just me and Ellison in the last lap. I kind of slipped up on him after the bell and when we got to the last straight I pulled the trigger. For a second I didn't think anything was going to happen. Then it caught and I blew by him. I actually ended up getting him by seven, but he probably eased off when he saw I wasn't going to come back to him. Bruce was beside himself. I think he has decided that he, you know, *discovered* me or something. Despite the fact that I had to run a 4:00.3 last year before he hardly said more than hello."

"How did his race go?"

"Oh, he just blew them right off the track. Art Dulong, Drayton, and that guy from Minnesota. They were never even in it. He ran 8:32 like it was a workout."

Mizner shook his head. "It would have been great to see. Both of you." But Cassidy knew what he was saying.

"So what is the word here? Is it confirmed?"

"Shit yes. They think maybe three, four months of no training. Even then it's touch and go because of the possibility of relapses. But at least I get out of here pretty soon."

"Well, hey, at least you didn't blow your eligibility. Except for cross-country." Very quietly, this last.

"Hey, listen. I already have a complete list of the silver linings. It's the goddamn cloud that's killing me."

"Yeah." Cassidy looked at his feet. There were no good words for this one, he thought. A runner who could not run was out of his element. He would not even think of himself as an athlete; ridiculously there would be a kind of guilt about it; that was the worst part. He would begin to feel uncomfortable around his training comrades and the feeling would be mutual, like a newly wounded soldier among the embarrassed whole ones, who would not wish to be reminded of certain roll-the-dice aspects of life. Cassidy was not surprised when Mizner told him he was going to move out of Doobey Hall for the next quarter. This was getting them both down. Mizner sensed it and changed the subject.

"What's happening with all the yelling and screaming on the haircut rules?"

"Hmmm. I wish I knew. It seems they are really serious about the thing. I hear they've been cracking down around Farley Hall, measuring sideburns with little rulers, making guys change shirts before they let them eat, stuff like that. Real, you know, brilliant stuff from the football minds over there. Even the football players are mad as hell. Nothing has happened at Doobey yet, but everyone figures they just haven't quite gotten around to us."

"Jeez. And me stuck in the infirmary."

"Consider yourself lucky. That goddamn Hosford volunteered my room for some kind of rabble-rousing meeting tonight." He looked at his watch irritably.

"I guess I'd better go. They might set fire to my Kip Keino poster or something." He tossed his beer can into the trash can and winced as it clanged. He had forgotten.

"Is there anything I can—"

"Naw. I've got everything; the guys brought my books and stuff. You better take off. Thanks for the pizza; I'd kiss you but . . ."

Cassidy laughed. "Then I'd catch it too and we could be roommates in here. Look, you take care of yourself, yuh hear? I know . . . I know, this is a pretty rough deal . . ."

"Well, the tour was getting to me a little, you know? I mean Akron one night, Utica the next. Now at least I can take the time to work on my steps and follow-through."

"And coming *over* the ball, don't forget to come over the ball . . ."

Mizner laughed. "No doubt. Hey Cass, really, congratulations on Millrose. I think it's just great. You should have heard me when I read the paper Saturday morning. They thought I had slipped and broken my ass on the way to the john or something." Cassidy nodded, smiled at him, and turned for the door just as it opened brusquely. The white-stockinged fireplug stood glaring at him.

"You!" she cried. Cassidy leaned over and solemnly kissed her on the forehead, then sprinted out the door dodging a relatively serious swat with her rolled-up *Cosmo*.

On the way back to Doobey, walking along with his hands

jammed in his pockets, away from the chilly evening, he was filled with loss and an off-brand of nostalgia for events that were supposed to become part of his past but now wouldn't at all. In the mind's special processes, a ten-mile run takes far longer than the sixty minutes reported by a grandfather clock. Such time, in fact, hardly exists at all in the real world; it is all out on the trail somewhere, and you only go back to it when you are out there.

He and Mize had been through two solid years of such regular time-warp escapes together. There was something different about that, something beyond friendship; they had a way of sharing pain, of transferring hurt back and forth, without the banality of words.

But now in the vague recesses of his mind, Cassidy detected deep and sinister rumblings; storm clouds that chilled the air but were not yet visible on the horizon.

And too, he did not do well with hospitals and infirmaries; repositories of laboratory smells, lethal-looking silverware; launching pads for flagging hopes . . .

16

New Territory

QUENTON CASSIDY had returned from his daily afternoon
visit to Mizner and now sat in his darkening room feeling
not so much despair as nerve-jangling emptiness. The scenery
was closing in on him. Low blood pH, he thought; the trick is to
keep from getting nervous in the pack, like Bruce says. Think of
how anchovies must swim a thousand to a square yard with a
perfect twin on either side and a tiny bung flitting up ahead.

The *Kernsville Sun* lay in a heap at the foot of the bed. He had
stopped trying to read when the sun got too low and he realized
he was too tired to get up and turn on the light. So he just sat,
staring out the window. It was slim pickings in the limp little
sheet anyway; warmed-over wire stories, a hard-hitting editorial
on sewage bonds, an irate letter from a lady complaining about a
neighbor's dog shitting in her azaleas, and sports editor Jack

Hairlepp's column urging full support for Dick Doobey's next season. There was a quote from the coach about "some real fine junior college transfers who are going to be a real great help to us out there next year." At that point Cassidy had tossed the paper, idly wondering if Hairlepp drew his salary from the newspaper or just picked up his check on Friday from the athletic department's publicity office.

Perhaps he was too hard on the local gazette. There was, after all, real news in the human-interest vein on page 2A under the "Smile for the Day" logo. It seems that somewhere out in the great American night a felonious ebony hand had skillfully slid a flat piece of steel down a car window, allowing a hopped-up connoisseur of spot remover to become the temporary (if illegal) bailee of a Ford Fairlane with transmission problems; thrown into the deal was a dark green garbage bag in the backseat, the contents of which were exactly: someone's dead mother-in-law.

Cassidy had thought: *oh, this is a fun-loving citizenry.*

"HEY, how come it's so dark in here?" Hosford wandered in, cracking his knee on the edge of the dresser.

"I'm afraid if I turn on a light I'll look in the mirror and see that I look as bad as I feel," Cassidy said, but not uncheerfully.

"Ah well. Mind if I sit down? Hey, the *Sun.* Anything in here?"

"As usual the only important message is contained in *Doonesbury.*"

"Well, as it happens, I bring news myself. I hope it's not bad. Western Union guy just brought it a few minutes ago. I thought you were asleep, so I signed for it."

"Telegram? Thanks, Hos . . ."

"I'll mosey along, I guess. Hey, listen . . ."

"Hey, this is open . . ."

". . . congratulations, Cass, all the guys think it's just great."

"All the . . . Hosford! Come back here, you nosy son of a bitch . . ."

"BRUCE? Sorry to call during dinner, but you'll never guess—"

"You got invited to the Sunkist Games next weekend," Denton said. Cassidy slumped.

"How the hell did you know?"

"I talked to the meet director when we were at Millrose."

"What did he say?"

"He wanted to know if I thought you could go under four minutes on his track in San Diego."

"And?"

"I asked him can a fish hold his breath under water."

Cassidy yelped, then calmed himself.

"Wonderful, Bruce. I haven't even run that outdoors yet . . ."

"Life is short, life is hard."

"You're running the three there?"

"Right."

"Good field?"

"I don't know what you call good. Just Shorter and a bunch of—"

"Shorter!"

"Mmmm. You'd think the little marathoner bastard would stick to the great outdoors. Unfortunately he seems to *like* the boards. And in case it slipped your mind, he once held the American record for two-mile indoors. On that very track."

"How, uh, do you think you'll handle him, Bruce?" Was that concern in his voice? Denton rattled around on his end for a few seconds; Cassidy couldn't tell what he was doing.

"Why, Quenton, *I'll break his back* . . ."

BRAGGADOCIO HAS LITTLE TO DO with it, however, when the really good boys clash and everyone is feeling chipper. The two gold medalists broke away from the field early and were soon circling the track at a distressing pace that quickly found most of the other runners lapped. Although Denton's credentials were in a race slightly longer than three miles and Shorter's in the marathon, their training was remarkably similar. The crowd was standing during the last half mile; the lead changed three times as they probed at each other. Denton's long powerful strides were matched by Shorter's clipped, silky ones. The marathoner was so smooth as to give the impression of gliding on wheels. The strain of the pace showed around the edges of their otherwise unemotional faces. Cassidy watched in awe as they threw surges at each other. *Sheeeitfire,* Cassidy thought, this is awful. We need some relief.

His shouts were lost in the general pandemonium as the two runners entered the final lap with Denton slightly in front and Shorter on his outside shoulder. Cassidy figured it was highly unlikely that a marathoner would be able to outsprint a 5000-meter champion, but his joyous victory whoop came just a trifle too early. It was a doubly painful revelation to watch the all-too-clear demonstration of mortality that was the last lap of that race. Frank Shorter had to break an American indoor record for three miles, and his margin of victory was exactly one tenth of a second, but there was no doubt whatsoever that when Bruce Denton reached the finish line, he had the unique experience of finding the yarn already parted for him. Cassidy was stunned.

Despite the incredible effort of their contest, the two runners were soon coherent enough to be interviewed by a particularly irrelevant Howard Cosell. Cassidy waited outside the glow of hot television lights in a pale haze of his own confusion. He had never seen Denton lose a race and he wasn't sure yet how he felt. When the interview was over, Denton and Shorter left the infield together and sprinted through a veritable tidal wave of little kids waving programs and pens. Denton turned, spotted Cassidy, motioned for him to join them. When the miler caught up to the pair of distance men in the hallway, they were already lost in the numerical shorthand of training talk. Shorter was reserved, shy, yet with a sweetness that seemed positively contrary to the aggression he summoned up for his competitors. His eyes reflected that irony. Cassidy wanted to ask him a hundred questions, but he bit his tongue. He was in truth a bit flabbergasted. First he had watched Denton outsprinted by a marathoner and now he and that marathoner were jogging along chatting about training like it was old home week. Denton had never mentioned that he even knew Shorter. Cassidy only half listened to the mumble of mileage figures:

". . . at altitude of course, and then 123, 132, 137, and 145, but with only two interval sessions a week . . ." ". . . and a long one on Sunday, about 20, Louise goes the first 10 with us . . ." ". . . step-down starting with a 4:12 mile and a 3:02 three quarters . . ." ". . . then 35 times 220 all of them pretty quick for me, 28 to 30 or so . . ." And so on. It was quiet for several seconds before he realized he had been spoken to.

"I'm sorry?" Cassidy said.

"I said Millrose. You won Millrose two weeks ago, didn't you?" Shorter was being polite, trying to include him in the conversation.

"Ah. Yes. The field wasn't that strong, you see . . ."

"Well, anyone who can run close to four on that track gets my respect. I think they made it out of pound cake dyed green."

"At least no one will get shin splints on the thing."

"I hate to interrupt a medical discussion," Denton said, pointing to a clock on the wall, "but I believe it's time for the stud milers among us to be doing some striders. This is one meet they generally manage to run on time. Mr. Shorter here finished the three so quickly he put them several minutes ahead."

Cassidy held out his hand to Shorter. "Hey, it was nice to

meet you. Uh, do you have any parting words for an aspiring young runner?"

Shorter looked puzzled, amused. He looked over at Denton, then smiled back at Cassidy.

"Well, no, not actually. Except have a good time."

Denton laughed and waved Cassidy off.

"That one," Denton said, tilting his head at the departing miler. "Keep your eye on that one . . ."

Shorter nodded.

THAT NIGHT Quenton Cassidy ran the best mile of his life and thereby changed his position in the tiny universe of runners nearly imperceptibly. He ran 4:00.1 and of course would never be quite the same. But his race was also a different kind of revelation.

And although Denton tried several times on the flight back to put things into perspective for him, Cassidy knew he was on the fearful and nebulous border of new territory.

He finished fifth, and was lucky to get that.

17

Breaking Down

CASSIDY HAD BEEN THROUGH IT BEFORE, every one of them had at one time or another, but it had never been quite this bad. Denton called it "breaking down," although Cassidy preferred the nomenclature of certain Caribbean quasi-religious groups; walking death was much closer to it. Quite a bit more, really, than the simple exhaustion of a single difficult workout, breaking down was a cumulative physical morbidity that usually built up over several weeks and left the runner struggling to recover from one session to the next.

The object, according to Denton, was to "run through" the thing, just as he maintained one should attempt to "run through" most of those other little hubcaps life rolls into your lane; everything from death in the family to cancer of the colon.

Breaking down was not a required checkpoint on the road to

competitive fitness. In fact, many coaches warned against it. But Denton viewed it as an opportunity to leapfrog over months of safer, less strenuous training, thus tempering survival-hardened muscles. The alternative, total rest, was too much the other extreme, the easy way out. That wouldn't do.

The toll on the runner—and those around him—was high, psychologically as well as physically. He became weak, depressed; he needed twelve to fourteen hours of sleep a night. He was literally desperate for rest, spent his waking hours with his legs elevated, in a state of general irritability. He became asexual, rendered, in the words of the immortal limerick, really quite useless on dates. He was a thoroughly unpleasant person.

But then his life was most certainly focused on the Task. And hadn't he decided at one time that he would do whatever was necessary to become . . . whatever it was he could become? Perhaps. But at this juncture, many a runner begins to reexamine some of the previously unexamined premises. The question that plagues the runner undergoing breakdown training is: Why Am I Living Like This? The question eventually becomes: Is This Living?

From the crucible of such inner turmoil come the various metals, soft or brittle, flawed or pure, precious or common, that determine the good runners, the great runners, and perhaps the former runners. For those who cannot deal with (or evade) the consequences of their singular objective will simply fade away from it all and go on to less arduous pursuits. There has probably never been one yet who has done so, however, without leaving a part of himself there in the quiet tiled solace of the early afternoon locker room, knotting his loathsome-smelling laces for yet another, Jesus God, ten-miler with the boys. Once a runner . . .

Cassidy always felt that those who partook of the difficult pleasures of the highly competitive runner only when comfortable, when in a state of high energy, when rested, elated, or untroubled by previous exertions, such dilettantes missed the point. They were the ones who showed up at the beginning of the season, perhaps hung on for a few rough periods, maybe ran a race or two. But Cassidy noticed that their eyes always gave them away; the gloom, one could tell, was too much for them. It would soon engulf them. They would begin to ask themselves the Questions too many times. Soon they would miss a workout. Then a few in a row. Then they would chicken out on themselves during the tough, stupid, endless middle of a bad race. And you don't easily hide such things from yourself, much less your teammates. Soon when the questions were posed, there would be no answers. The runner would begin to feel self-conscious around the others, knowing that he was no longer one of them; eventually he would drift off, and be a runner no more . . .

Quenton Cassidy's method of dealing with fundamental doubts was simple: he didn't think about them at all. These questions had been considered a long time ago, decisions made, answers recorded, and the book closed. If it had to be reopened every time the going got rough, he would spend more time rationalizing than training; his log would start to disclose embarrassing information, perhaps blank squares. Even a self-made obsessive-compulsive could not tolerate that. He was uninterested in the perspective of the fringe runners, the philosopher runners, the training rats; those who sat around reading abstruse and meaningless articles in *Runner's World*, coining yet more phrases to describe the indescribable, waxing mystical over the various states of euphoria that the anointed were allegedly privy to.

On the track, the Cassidys of the world ate such specimens alive.

Cassidy sought no euphoric interludes. They came, when they did, quite naturally and he was content to enjoy them privately. He ran not for crypto-religious reasons, but to win races, to cover ground fast. Not only to be better than his fellows, but better than himself. To be faster by a tenth of a second, by an inch, by two feet or two yards, than he had been the week or year before. He sought to conquer the physical limitations placed upon him by a three-dimensional world (and if Time is the fourth dimension, that too was his province). If he could conquer the weakness, the cowardice in himself, he would not worry about the rest; it would come. Training was a rite of purification; from it came speed, strength. Racing was a rite of death; from it came knowledge. Such rites demand, if they are to be meaningful at all, a certain amount of time spent precisely on the Red Line, where you can lean over the manicured putting green at the edge of the precipice and see exactly nothing.

Anything else that comes out of that process was by-product. Certain compliments and observations made him uneasy; he explained that he was just a runner; an athlete, really, with an absurdly difficult task. He was not a health nut, was not out to mold himself a stylishly slim body. He did not live on nuts and berries; if the furnace was hot enough, anything would burn, even Big Macs. He listened carefully to his body and heeded strange requests. Like a pregnant woman, he sometimes sought artichoke hearts, pickled beets, smoked oysters. His daily toil was arduous; satisfying on the whole, but not the bounding, joyous nature romp described in the magazines. Other runners, *real* runners, understood it quite well.

Quenton Cassidy knew what the mystic-runners, the joggers, the runner-poets, the Zen runners, and others of their ilk were talking about. But he also knew that their euphoric selves were generally nowhere to be seen on dark, rainy mornings. They primarily wanted to talk it, not do it. Cassidy very early on understood that a true runner ran even when he didn't feel like it, and raced when he was supposed to, without excuses and with nothing held back. He ran to win, would die in the process if necessary, and was unimpressed by those who disavowed such a base motivation. You are not allowed to renounce that which you never possessed, he thought.

The true competitive runner, simmering in his own existential juices, endured his melancholia the only way he knew how: gently, together with those few others who also endured it, yet very much alone. He ran because it grounded him in basics. There was both life and death in it; it was unadulterated by media hype, trivial cares, political meddling. He suspected it kept him from that most real variety of schizophrenia that the republic was then sprouting like mushrooms on a stump.

Running to him was real; the way he did it the realest thing he knew. It was all joy and woe, hard as diamond; it made him weary beyond comprehension. But it also made him free.

18.
Meetings

SITTING QUIETLY over his sandwiches, Cassidy chewed mechanically. He did not look happy. From the kitchen came metallic clatter and laughter; cooks, he thought, are a carefree lot after everyone has been fed.

This morning had been typical of the past two weeks. Cassidy wondered quite seriously if he could (should someone put a big gun to his head) go out on the track and run a 4:30 mile flat out. The morning seven had been sluggish and Mize wasn't there to commiserate with. While dressing for his first class he glanced at the mirror, shrugged, went back to bed. He slept soundly for five hours, woke grumpily, and stumbled downstairs for a late lunch. In the three weeks since the Sunkist meet Denton had taken a special interest in his training. They now ran together in the afternoons, an arrangement approved by Cornwall since Cassidy's growing strength was beginning to dishearten the others in interval workouts.

Denton then insisted on raising mileage. Tired as he was after the Sunkist weekend, Monday was a twenty-three-mile day. The week totaled 127 and it appeared they would not be slacking off any. He lived from workout to workout, hanging on like a crazed marsupial on a branch in a flash flood. Life was becoming, he admitted to himself, more than a little morbid.

Hosford wandered over with his tray.

"Sandwiches again," he said, sitting down heavily across from Cassidy.

"Fuel for the furnace, hardly makes any difference," Cassidy said. To demonstrate his point, perhaps, he chewed as if it were an effort he could barely maintain.

"Are you going to run Boston Garden this weekend? Cornwall says that if you want to double, he might take a two-mile relay."

"I'm not even sure I can run the mile. The way I've been drag-assing around here for two weeks, I may have to take up triple jumping or something."

"Well, just a thought. I suppose you heard about Pospicil?"

"Hosford, I've been underwater for two weeks. What about Pospicil?"

"That asshole Slattery gave him a pretty hard time yesterday. Came up to him at the training table at Farley and started flipping at his hair, you know, real nasty like, saying stuff like, 'Don't you know this is the training table, deary? Where the athletes eat—men athletes, honey, not girls . . .' That kind of stuff. About as bad as it could be."

"Aw, Christ. Poss probably didn't understand their idiot rules in the first place. He doesn't even speak much regular English, much less grit English."

"I don't think he knew anything about it. How would you like to be the number three player in your country, get a big recruiting come-on, show up in the wonderful United States of America with your tennis racket and a big smile, and then run into an ass-hole like Slattery with his haircut rules? I bet Poss has never even *seen* a redneck before. Jeez, poor guy."

"When you think of the crap that Slattery pulled when he was an undergraduate here . . ." Cassidy shook his head.

"Uh, look, what I really wanted to tell you was that some of the tennis guys got pretty hot about the whole thing. And they got some of the track guys stirred up again. I mean, they all re-spect your opinion and all, especially that stuff about living well being the best revenge, but I think maybe it's gone too far now."

"And?"

"Bottom line is there's another meeting in your room to-night."

"My room?"

"I guess that was my fault. I told them you probably wouldn't mind. Plus everyone knows that you're planning to go to law school and all that. They listen to you, Cass."

Cassidy said nothing, rubbed his eyes painfully.

"Cass, somebody has got to do something. This Pospicil thing is not the first. People are starting to get pretty upset, even a bunch of football guys. I mean, you being a team captain and all, it's really kind of your job—"

"Okay, okay, Hos*ford*! Christ, one hundred thirty-two miles last week, Mize flat on his ass, Andrea in some kind of snit, Den-ton's intervals got me walking around bumping into walls, and now suddenly the entire football staff is on the warpath." He rubbed his eyes again, and Hosford for a horrifying moment thought he was going to blubber.

"Look, Hos, I'll come and listen," Cassidy said. "Maybe there is some reasonable course of action to take. But I get this gut feeling . . ."

"Not too hopeful, huh?"

"Hosford, you're talking Southern football mentality now. People who covered five thousand square yards of beautiful cool stadium grass with a green plastic death mat that scrapes big hunks of skin off your ass if you so much as sit down on it wrong. People who think Joe Paterno is a dangerous intellectual. People who think Vietnam is a . . . an *opportunity*. I mean, how are you gonna . . ." This was just making him tired. Hosford didn't really understand what they were dealing with yet. Cassidy tossed his sandwich on the tray like a blackjack dealer disinterestedly busting himself.

Hosford would have liked to have snickered at the death mat stuff, but knew better. Cassidy picked up his tray, deposited it on the cart with a clatter, and wandered out of the dining room feeling perhaps as bleak a child of America as the tots on the Appalachia posters. Quenton Cassidy reflected upon the fact that at least he was well fed.

He knew though that had a single germ strolled up and surveyed the premises, it could have moved in without even a damage deposit. This is definitely a low ebb, he thought. He stood at the bottom of the stairs, looking tiredly out through the living room to the front yard where two dogs fought without enthusiasm for a small patch of shade. At times like this he felt weary and land-bound, and soothed himself by thinking of the ocean. He pictured translucent pink anemones, floating like ladies with deadly long skirts. Then: a cero mackerel somewhere on the pale turquoise of the Bahama Bank working a school of greenies with unemotional fervor; a guide poles the flats soundlessly, turns wrinkled black cheeks to the burning sun, and smiles to visions of Canadian schoolteachers "on holiday."

Cassidy did not look forward to this gathering of irate citizens in his room, but tomorrow night he was taking Andrea to the Winjammer and that, along with his sea thoughts, would get him through another day. Still, it became in the end a little difficult making it up the three flights of stairs back to the musky womb of his bed.

19.

The Awesome Midnight Raid

THE WINJAMMER would have at one time been called "camp," with multicolored lights and unlikely looking plastic fruit hanging about. There was a pleasant little trio that sounded not unlike the Pozo-Seco Singers, but for Cassidy the real allure was the raw Apalachicola oysters, offered at $1.50 per dozen and, of course, the draft beer, which was very cold.

They were due for a "talk" of some kind, he and Andrea, but Cassidy was not very good at "talks" and could not remember one that did not end in some kind of confusing nastiness; abstract dialogue from a Woody Allen screenplay without enough detachment to make it funny.

Instead, he made much over the oysters, mixing horseradish in his cocktail sauce and adding a dash of Tabasco. And he told her of the dire rumblings around Doobey Hall.

"It seems I have become the official draftsman. It was my own fault, of course. I told them that their petition was too prolix. That impressed them so much that I found myself at the typewriter with everyone talking at once."

"So what happens now?"

"Well, nothing maybe. We got something whipped into shape, but we sat around talking for a while and everyone agreed to hold off again and see if maybe the thing won't just blow over. Hell, we're athletes; we don't need this kind of aggravation. But if things keep up, they will take the petitions around and see how many signatures they can get on them. If we have enough support among the rest of the teams, they will take them to the athletic department and then it's their move."

"Do you think it will do any good?"

"Oh, yes, petitioning Dick Doobey and the athletic department will be like going down to the Kissimmee Zoo and formally debating the cotton-top marmoset. It will win the day, I'm sure of it."

"Quenton."

"Wanta dance?"

"If you do."

Cassidy had a helpless affinity for places like the Winjammer. In a room off to the side, two long-haired construction workers clomped around the pool table in their heavy boots, obviously stoned into yesterday, laughing at each other's ineptness.

"Goddamn, Harlan," said one as a ball jumped the rail and hit the wall with a crack, "put some power to it. You ain't got a black hair on your ass 'less you dent some paneling." They both keeled over, helpless in the face of each other's wit.

Cassidy thought: *oh, to be blue collar in America in the seventies. Real life, such as it is, is being committed here.*

"Andrea, do you know this is the first time I have touched your body with any sort of lust in mind in four days?"

"I know." Of course she knew, Cassidy thought, such time-tables are a lady's tea and scones.

"I wonder why that might be."

"Well, there was the organic test on Monday, there was that awful computer program that wouldn't run, there is the fact that you are becoming a very difficult person to get along with . . ."

"Ah . . ."

"Quenton, I'm trying very hard to understand, really, but what can possibly justify what you are doing to yourself? You've started cutting classes, you can't eat dinner because you're still tied up in knots, you fall asleep over your books after fifteen minutes of studying . . ."

"Andrea, this is not a permanent condition you are seeing here. Bruce says—"

"Bruce says, Bruce says."

"Isn't this getting a little obvious now?"

"Oh, Quenton, I wonder sometimes if you know how I really feel about you. How much I'd like for it to work out. If there was only some compromise, some—"

"Well, there you have touched upon something, Andrea, because that's it right there: the thing itself is the absence of compromise. There are no . . . deals available. I wish there was some way to explain that. The thing . . . doesn't dilute."

He shrugged and held her closer. Just trying to explain was tiring. You can either do it or not do it, he thought, but you can't talk about it worth a damn. "Let's not discuss it any-more," she said. "The more we talk the more it slips away." The music stopped but they lingered, still holding each other closely. It was true; he did not have the ability to give that which she most needed, and she did not have the ability to understand that eerie dimension to him that even he did not know well. These fundamental imbalances led them into con-centric circles of ever decreasing size: a nautilus shell of their discontent.

ℒ

THE AWESOME MIDNIGHT RAID took place that night. It started as a low rumble on the first floor, as if a group of rowdies were just getting in from their rounds. But instead of gradually calming down, the rumble soon became a roar. Cassidy awoke dreamlike to the racket. There seemed to be loud arguments, much scuffling about, objects hitting walls, random bellows in the night. When he was finally completely awake, he sat up and listened carefully. There was no laughter or mirth of any kind in the tumult, but there were definite traces of panic and anger. The resident counselor had gone early for the weekend, leaving the three team captains technically in charge, so Cassidy jumped up and pulled on some clothes.

What was happening below was that Harold Slattery and two other assistant football coaches were, very simply, raiding the dormitory. They were aware that members of the opposite sex occasionally spent the night at Doobey, and it was their intent to ferret out the transgressors and perhaps have some fun in the bargain. They were going through the rooms, one by one, knocking once loudly and then barging in with their flashlights, invoking their unassailable authority:

"Coaches! Coming in!" Then they rushed into the room. Those athletes who fortuitously found themselves sleeping alone heard them say something like: "This one's clean. Mark 'im off." Then they tromped off to the next room, hoping for some kind of action. Soon they had an entourage of irate athletes following along behind them, grumbling, shouting, and perhaps on the verge of forming a lynching party, authority or no.

Cassidy was almost out the door when he heard the tumult come to a sudden halt below. The coaches had reached room 207 and, self-righteousness and bravado running high, had decided to forgo the knock as being too polite and simply barge in. When they got inside, they found themselves staring into the small, dark, and very genuine-looking hole which was the muzzle of Jack Nubbins's .45. In the dim light it barked deafeningly and the doorknob, only a few inches from Harold Slattery's hand, disappeared with a sharp metallic clang.

Nubbins switched on the light sleepily, the gun still trained on the wide-eyed Slattery. Betty Sue huddled up under the blanket, her tiny frightened green eyes peering out.

"I'm not that good a shot," Nubbins said, yawning. "I might have blowed your dinner away!" Slattery stood still as a snapshot, his upper lip white with that most absolute brand of fear you get right before your life flashes in front of your eyes. It was probably the yawn that made the little fuzzy hairs stand up on the back of his thick neck.

"Now I will generally hit a shot like that, mind, but right about now I am sleepy-eyed. Lot of good shots will wake up from a sound sleep and not be able to hit a blessed thing . . ."

"We're uh . . ."

"Yeah, I know what you are," Nubbins said calmly. "But be goddamned if I didn't think you was a ordinary burglar. Didn't you think so, Betty Sue?" He looked over at the frightened girl, who didn't so much as blink. "Yeah, I did too, honey. Matter of fact, he might still be a burglar for all I know. I can't see real well in this here light."

"Now look here, Nubbins . . ." Slattery was regaining some of his composure and did not like the idea of this anecdote getting around. It was time to recoup himself a little dignity and he took one nearly imperceptible step forward as he spoke. The gun exploded again and the molding on the opposite side of the door frame splattered.

"There I go again," said Nubbins. "I was actually aiming about three inches higher than that." By the time the plaster and wood chips had settled, Slattery and his gang had formally abandoned the hunt.

When Cassidy got to the second floor it was all over. Everyone was talking at once and no one was making any sense. Once he got the story pieced together it occurred to him that some truly dark forces, ignorant of their own madness, were at work.

And fate, of course, swings to and fro on tiny hinges; a cable is misplaced and a king assassinated; a vacuum tube blinks and a ship is lost with all hands; a general fails to get laid and thousands are firebombed . . .

20.

Night Run

CASSIDY RACED ALONG to a night rhythm, *pocketa-pocketa*, a steady tattoo of pleasant solitary effort that starred him under many streetlights, rendered him anonymous in dark neighborhoods, sent him smoothly up and down the gentle hills of Kernsville while dogs howled and Mom and Pop passed the mashed potatoes.

A passerby might have thought him in a trance, but he missed nothing in his darkling backdrop: the smells of winter-blooming flowers, clean coolness of blackjack oak, damp pepper of Spanish moss. The sounds were of early-evening TV silliness, dinner, children's squabbles. He was a shaded meteor plumbing a twinkling universe. The night made even more acute the runner's senses, lent more poignancy to his aloneness, made his fast pace seem even faster, generated an urgency, a subdued excitement in the act of solitary motion.

The seamless sphere of his reverie was occasionally marred by some cretin in a Chevrolet who would yell: "Hey Runner Runner!" Cassidy would flip a finger reflexively and otherwise indicate his displeasure by some epithet. For years he had tried ignoring them to no effect. Now his policy was to lash back. They were surprised when the runner (a gentle creature, no?) would exhibit such aggressiveness. What it was in human nature that generated this irresistible urge to bait a runner, he did not know. But he knew by now that it was deep, formidable, and nearly universal. An English writer of a different era recorded the taunts of street urchins: "Hey, looke at the runner, ee's got nae clothes on!" Some threw things. At Cassidy some would yell "hut, two, three, four . . ." and laugh at their own preposterous wit, unable to disassociate running from the military experience.

Once, by sprinting nearly two hundred yards, he caught up to a particularly obnoxious carload of rowdies who, panic-stricken now, were halted at an uncooperative red light. Thinking themselves safe after rolling up the windows and locking the doors, they watched in horror as Cassidy ran up the trunk and over the top of the car without breaking stride.

In training he was fearless, felt himself too easily capable of violence. He often contemplated what he would do if someone stopped and challenged him. He figured he would put them through a little of what his life was all about first; taunt them into giving chase. He would stay just a little out of their grasp, egg them on and on. Perhaps they would make half a mile or so, depending on how well he could lure them; perhaps their own sense of pride might surface, a by-product of a terrible misconception about what was actually happening. Shorter had once run the legs off an entire gang of hooligans in the hills of New

Mexico, despite already being tired from a fifteen-mile run. You would watch for the signs, Cassidy thought, the ones you knew so well; the pain, the bewilderment, the blankness that would eventually come close to despair. He would make it a challenge, so they would forget their original purpose and keep on going just to show this bastard, this . . . this . . . (then it would dawn on them) *runner.*

Then he would simply turn and face them. He would take on anyone like that, he thought. He would take on Muhammad Ali, so long as he could direct the preliminaries.

Cassidy knew very well that he could take men, otherwise strong and brave men, to places they had never been before. Places where life and death overlapped in surreal valleys of muscle gloom and heart despair, where one begins to realize once more that nothing really matters at all and that stopping (death?) is all; where all men finally get the slick skin of civilization off and see that soft pink glow inside that tells you—in both cunnilingus and bullet wounds—*that there are no secrets.*

A visitor's taste, in short, of the distance runner's daily fare. He would fight them then, if they still wanted to, after they knew. But they wouldn't want to, he was sure of that. They would walk away with nothing more than a hard-won understanding.

This night no one stopped. No one gave form to verbal menace. No one did any more than add his simpleminded bleating to the dark background of the runner's ritual.

Cassidy flew through the night.

"BRUCE," he said into the telephone, "I need to talk to you. I'm at Doobey now and I can't talk on this hall phone. Can you meet me at the Nineties or something?"

"Sure. Where have you been? I thought you were going to do quarters with me this afternoon. Did you run?"

"Of course I ran. I just did ten hard. Listen, I had to go see

Dick Doobey in his office this afternoon. Something's up. Can you meet me there in fifteen minutes or so?"

"Okay. But I'm not going to sit there drinking beer all night like you guys. I'll have a couple and—"

"Okay, okay. No problem. I gotta take a shower, just got in. See you there."

THE NINETIES was not crowded during the middle of the week; Fat Fred, the owner, was so exultant having Bruce Denton in his place that he bought him a pitcher of beer. It was an enthusiasm he felt he could afford, there being a relative dearth of gold medal winners in Kernsville. The two runners retreated to a corner booth.

"So what is the crisis?" Denton was pouring as the jukebox held forth: "... *and time ... washes clean ... lu-huv's wounds unseen ...*"

"You've seen the stuff in the papers this morning?"

"Who hasn't?"

"Well, they have decided that since I was the one who typed up the petition and also the one who delivered the signatures to the A.D., that this whole thing was conceived and, uh, '*per*petrated' as they say, by myself and one or two other unnamed conspirators."

"How do they figure? Every jock in this school is so pissed off ..."

"I'm convinced they really are as fucking stupid as they seem. When they couldn't find themselves an outside agitator—"

"Jeez, the whole thing looked pretty mild to me."

"You would think. But Doobey sat there and told me he didn't really blame me for all this fuss. He figures the real blame should be leveled at all the communist and left-leaning professors on the other side of the campus who have been working on my poor little brain all these years."

"Good God. Do you suppose he's serious?"

"Oh, he's serious all right. He isn't a humorous man. He kept coming up with all these military analogies. 'In the army, by God, you did what you were told, or they broke your plate—over your head.' That kind of thing. And then he goes into this stuff about my professors. Christ! Here I've been taught by fuel-injected right-wing loonies and closet Nazis for three years and that idiot thinks I've been brainwashed by some leftist academic conspiracy. My goddamn econ teacher thinks Milton Friedman is a liberal! Hell, if this campus got a decent teacher, they'd have the son of a bitch rebinding books behind the stacks somewhere . . ."

"All right, calm down. What happened exactly?"

Cassidy finished his second glass with a grimace. He was still dehydrated from the run.

"They're taking a hard line. Apparently what's got everyone all stirred up is the fact that a bunch of football players signed the damned thing. Apparently Doobey was called on the carpet by Prigman himself about it. I guess if it weren't for the football players involved, they could probably just write the thing off by saying the spring sports guys have gone commie on us. You know, we're all in individual events anyway, not part of, you know, a team effort . . ."

"Oh say, that makes sense . . ."

"And I think I'm beginning to get wind of a little gambit that smells something like the bottom of somebody's locker."

"Lively analogy." The jukebox played: ". . . *has anybody here seen sweet thang . . .*"

"Doobey said something to the effect that he figured something like this was going on during the football season, otherwise with the talent they had, they would have never gone four and six. Get the drift?"

"What!" Denton was incredulous. "They're gonna try and pin their lousy football season . . ."

Cassidy let the air out of his lungs. Physically he was keen, immensely strong at this point in his life; he could run a hundred miles. Yet he was starting to feel a smothering weight descending over him, a pale shroud he was helpless to evade.

I feel old, he thought. I have been dead once, I guess you can't get any older than that. But that was long ago, in the salt salt sea.

To Denton, still sitting looking unbelieving at the ceiling, he said: "Bruce, I'm so close. It seems so stupid to have something like this . . ."

"Yes. I know, but hang tough, don't get nervous in the pack . . ."

THREE DAYS LATER, a befuddled Coach Cornwall called Cassidy into his office and told him that due to circumstances over which he, as track coach, had no control, Quenton Cassidy would be henceforth suspended from participation in intercollegiate athletics.

21.

Steven C. Prigman

SOUTHEASTERN UNIVERSITY President Steven C. Prigman had once sat on the Florida Supreme Court bench and during his seven-year tenure had taken part in several illustrious decisions that stood as landmarks of jurisprudential comedy.

The most famous of these much-read cases involved a young black man who had the audacity to request admission to Southeastern University's law school. He wasn't exactly turned down, but they did lose his application. The third time they lost it, he filed suit and was quickly hooted out of state circuit court. From there he took his appeal to the august tribunal upon which sat His Honor Justice Prigman and six of his toadies. Taking scant time to deliberate after oral arguments, they came down with a decision that said, in so many words, that if God Almighty had wanted all races to go to white law schools,

Negroes would have been born with perfect LSAT scores and calfskin briefcases. Some months later, the United States Supreme Court, ignoring entirely the interesting logic used to arrive at the lower-court decision, overturned the case at the same time it issued its *Brown v. Board of Education* ruling, and sent it back to Justice Prigman and company without so much as a "nice try."

At this point the justices showed some real imagination. Declaring that the U.S. Supreme Court had made its determination on "constitutional grounds" alone, they decided that if there were other considerations for keeping the black man out, then the decision wouldn't apply. Therefore, they decided to appoint a local circuit judge to be a "special master" to make a study of the situation and find out what would happen were a black man to enter the law school. The "special master" quickly found out that all hell would, of course, break loose; this would take the form of mass student withdrawals and attendant financial collapse. There would be great pandemonium in the school itself: riots, vandalism, even food fights. The "special master" was able to intuit these dire consequences by the tried-and-true interview method ("Are you going to riot?" "Of course!" "Okay.").

And so it was that the Honorable Florida Supreme Court was able, in all good conscience, to blatantly disobey a direct mandate of the United States Supreme Court by saying that their new ruling denied admission to the student not on constitutional grounds, but on the inherent police power of the government to prevent violence. That the said violence would be caused by law-breaking (and perhaps imaginary) whites, concerned them not a whit. The young black man, out of money and patience, disgustedly threw in the towel and went north to procure his degree.

Steven C. Prigman had always been a charter member of the Florida Panhandle good old boy network. Sipping fifteen-year-old bourbon, his handsome ruddy face aglow with good humor, he could charm the fangs off water moccasins. Although Sidecar Doobey often referred to him as a "snub-nose little twerp," the two men understood each other very well. Doobey was influential in helping Prigman relocate to an academic setting when the jurist decided to step down from the bench.

And when he finally did so, he left Tallahassee with no small measure of pride that he and his associates had been able, for even a short period of time, to stanch the flow of the twentieth century. Their golden moment, still preserved in volume 93 of the second *Southern Reporter* series, to this day provides many hours of comic relief for law students all across the country.

DICK DOOBEY had felt a trifle ill at ease the day before on his way to Prigman's office. His squishy, ripple-soled coaching shoes squeaked embarrassingly as he walked up the marble steps to the president's office.

"Hello, Roberta." He winked at the middle-aged and not unattractive brunette, wondering if the old man was getting any. She looked up pleasantly, greeted him, and then ushered him into the quiet office. She was a charming woman, but Doobey knew she did not like him. Her smile was that of a headwaiter.

"Well, Coach!" said the old man heartily, rising to shake hands. "Have a seat, my boy. Make yourself comfortable." In the battle of the giant offices, Prigman had it all over Dick Doobey, even though his carpet did not bear a giant Daryl the Swamp Dawg. It was decorated much more in the taste of a former state supreme court justice, the walls full of honorary degrees, hunting memorabilia, and photographs of Prigman with recognizable personages. Dick Doobey envied the dignified brown and tan hues that seemed to command much more respect than his colorful mishmash of caricatures and trophies. The aura of the office was, in a word, impressive, and Dick

Doobey never sat in that chair without feeling both fear and envy.

"Well, what kind of spring practice are we going to have this year?" Prigman asked. Doobey had not expected this kind of question, so frenzied had been his other problems of late. He started to launch into his routine about some junior college transfers and redshirts that were going to be "of real great help to us out there next year," but he didn't get very far before Prigman cut him off.

"Fine, fine. I know what some of our detractors are saying about last year's record, but I know you're going to pull the program together once you get your feet on the ground here."

"Well, yes sir, I feel that I'm just now getting to the point where I can—"

"Fine, fine. Coach, what I wanted to ask you about"—he reached over to a corner of his huge polished desk and held up a legal-sized xeroxed page—"is this. Do you know anything about it?"

Dick Doobey took the sheet, held it away from his face as if it were a small serpent, and studied it carefully. He tried to act as though he had never seen the likes before. Prigman knew better. At the top of the page was a paragraph that began: "We, the athletes of Southeastern University, hereby wish to make known certain grievances . . ." The page Doobey held contained thirty-eight signatures. There were other sheets as well, and Doobey knew that all in all, about 125 varsity athletes, including many of his own football players, had signed the petition.

"Well, sir, I do happen to know something about this particular matter."

"Perhaps you'd like to fill me in." There was the faintest hint of menace in the old man's voice.

"Well, sir, this morning an athlete from the track team dropped by a stack of these, uh, petitions, It seems that quite a few of the athletes have signed them and—"

"How many?"

"Well, sir, I don't know exactly but somewhere I would say, oh, around a hundred or so, sir, and—"

"A hundred!" He practically shouted it. Dick Doobey felt himself pressing backward in the soft chair.

"Well, yes sir, more or less, sir . . ."

"Any football men among 'em?"

"Oh, I don't know, sir, I didn't check the lists out very carefully or any—"

"I *asked* . . . if there were any football men . . . *on the lists?*" Very quietly, this last.

"Yes, sir! There were, oh, forty or so, I would say offhand, sir."

"Forty!" Prigman rested his chin on the steeple of his hands, turning his chair to the side, either deep in thought or too angry to speak. Doobey prayed to God it was the former.

The old man swung the chair back around and leaned forward, skewering Doobey against the chair with a stare that seemed a physical force. It was the kind of gesture Prigman had developed to a high art, and he noted with satisfaction Doobey's bobbing Adam's apple.

"Well, *Coach* Doobey, perhaps you can explain to me what in the devil all this is about?" Doobey started to say something but the old man continued.

"I mean, just for instance, what is this stuff about 'unwarranted neo-Gestapo raids upon athletes' rooms . . .' and 'militaristic hair and dress regulations . . .' Perhaps you could explain just what in the hell is happening on my campus, *Coach* Doobey!" He was half standing in front of his chair, but slowly forced himself to sit back down, giving the impression of rage brought under control only with great effort. Doobey had been thinking all morning what he would say right now and though he thought he had it worked out, it all left him now. He stared at the petition as if it would provide him with some clue.

"Well, Mr. President, it seems that some of the athletes are a little upset over our new hair and dress code, sir, and then there was an incident at the track dormitory the other night which was not authorized on my part and which perhaps was a little, uh, unwarranted, I mean, trying to be subjective about the whole thing and all . . ."

"What in the hell are you babbling about, man? What hair and dress code? What incident?"

"Well, sir, the code was a little idea of mine to try to boost morale a little, sir . . ."

Doobey filled in the old man as best he could. When he finished, the elder man sat sideways again, in deep thought. After a while, Doobey thought he had been forgotten such was the length of the old man's meditation. Finally, Prigman swung around to face Doobey, but he spoke so softly the coach had to lean forward to hear.

"I had a call from Walter Davis this morning. You know Walt?"

"Well, sir, I—"

"He's the UPI man out of Miami, Coach Doobey. But I couldn't talk to him right away because I had Norman Johnson on the other line. You know Norm?" Still very quiet.

"Yes, sir, I—"

"He's the AP man out of Miami. Well, it seems these representatives of our nation's wire services were pretty much interested in the same thing . . ." He held up the petition with one hand, tapping it briskly with the back of his other hand.

"The same thing as the fellow from *Sports Illustrated*—I've never had the pleasure of talking to those folks before—and the sports editors of about twelve or so major newspapers around the Southeast. Roberta has been real good about that. Anything with a circulation below fifty thousand and the call gets diverted to a vice president or a dean. Now, of course, I don't know how many calls *they* had . . ."

"I talked to quite a few myself and—"

"I'm not *interested!*"

"Yes, *sir!*"

"What I am interested in"—calmly now—"is exactly what in the name of all that's holy are we going to do about this thing now that you have so blithely gotten it rolling for us, *Coach* Doobey?"

"Well, I—"

"I mean, do you realize the implications, sir, of an athletes' revolt? Do you know, can you appreciate the fact that we've just gone through several years of strife and violence on our campuses because of our country's selfless battle against communism in Vietnam? And that throughout that time of crisis our athletes have been our mainstay, our rock? No matter what kind of crap was going on everywhere else, our boys were out there every Saturday, hitting hard, blocking clean, going at it like there was no tomorrow, giving it the old guts-balls *college try*. Why, those boys have been carrying on, in our darkest hour, our very *American traditions!*"

Doobey perked up. "Why, yes sir, that's exactly why—"

"I'm not *through*. And now, *Coach* Doobey, now just as our athletes had come to symbolize all that was good and loyal and patriotic about our country, now we find them running around and . . . and . . . *signing petitions!*"

"I'm as surprised as you are, sir!"

"Surprised *batshit!*" He picked up another sheet of paper. "'Sideburns not to be lower than a line extending perpendicular from the bottom tip of the earlobe . . .' Where did you get such . . . such *notions?*" His contempt was barely contained.

"Well, sir, some of them I picked up from my military training . . ."

"Mmmmmm."

". . . some of them were suggested by Assistant Coach Slattery, uh, he came up with the one about shirts with no collars . . ."

"Collars," said Prigman miserably.

". . . and some of them I just sort of made up myself, sir."

"Somehow I might have guessed that," said Prigman very softly to the ceiling.

THEIR CONFERENCE WENT ON into the afternoon. Prigman, his rage somewhat mollified, now concentrated on the logistics of the problem at hand. He pretty much knew what Doobey was going to tell him anyway, but was not about to forgo his pound of flesh. He would deal further with this dodo son of Sidecar's later; for the time being he was content to watch the involuntary quiver of fear that ran through the portly body every time he emphasized the word "coach." But this was a time for action; policy had to be formulated, the media had to be dealt with. It called for swift, clear, eminently intelligent decision making. It required, in short, the kind of grit that Prigman proudly reflected was precisely the reason he was where he was. Secretly, he relished the prospects.

"Who brought the petitions to your office?"

"It was a track man. A Quenton Cassidy, sir. He just dropped them off."

"Did he say anything when he left them?"

"Yes, sir. He told Mary Lou, that's my secretary, that he would be glad to talk the situation over with me at our mutual convenience."

"At your—"

"Mutual convenience, that's what he said, sir."

"Jesus H. Christ."

22.

Brady Grapehouse

Over the whirlpool in the large training room a hand-lettered sign read:

YOU CAN'T MAKE THE CLUB
SITTING IN THE TUB

Brady Grapehouse presided here and since he knew that healing waters sometimes had not so much to do with real physical injuries as with providing a good place to hide from a hurtful world, the sign—like everything else in this domain—was his idea.

He had been the head trainer at Southeastern for ten years before Dick Doobey arrived as football coach. Many generations of athletes felt a single emotion for Brady: love, pure and unabashed. If an interrogator were to corner the toughest, meanest son of a bitch of a lineman from among Brady's former customers and ask him point-blank if he loved Brady Grapehouse, the lineman would say: "Goddamn right I love Brady Grapehouse. *Everybody* loves Brady Grapehouse." Everybody except Dick Doobey, who hated Brady Grapehouse.

It was probably the love he generated among his athletes that did Brady in; everyone knew that Dick Doobey had told him his contract would not be renewed in order to bring in Zip Simmons, a sycophantic dolt Doobey knew from the army, whom he liked having around because he was one of the few grown-ups Doobey had ever been around who didn't make him feel at least a little dim-witted.

Like many men who found competence puzzling, Doobey did not like to have much of it around him at any one time.

Brady was nearly a caricature of himself. Short and round, he always had a cold stump of a cigar in his mouth (there was speculation he bought them that way from some furtive supplier). He had short wavy black hair flecked with gray; he gave the impression not so much of age as of having been around. He moved around the training room gracefully on the balls of his feet like the old boxer he was. Had he been in the service, he would have been the tough old top sergeant who everyone would admit, when cross-eyed drunk, was a pretty good son of a bitch.

Brady had seen them all. Hotshot all-American quarterbacks, hostile giant linemen, seven-foot basketball freaks, flashy tennis stars, future pro golfers—some of whom would make millions with their incredible legs, hands, and eyes. All of these were mixed in with the myriad ranks of steady performers, who were (though they didn't realize it at all) at the pinnacle of a life destined to peak so early that the rest of their lives would be a wistful reminiscence of days when poetic deeds were the order of the day.

Brady ministered to them all with the same gruff efficiency.

They would come to him, at times when they were physically quite well, tapping on the glass partition of his fishbowl office in the training room, usually in the morning when there was no taping going on and the place was a cool, tiled retreat.

"Uh, Brade," they would say, a little hangdog, "Brade, you gotta secont?"

"Gotta secont? Gotta secont? Now what else would I have better to do than sit around here jawboning with one of you jacklegs all mornin'?" The door would close and he would take it on. He was an uncle, priest, medical advisor, psychiatrist. They came to him with things they couldn't discuss with their closest friends. The married ones, cut off from the rough intimacy of the athletic bachelorhood, came in to talk about problems of the hearth: children, sex, fidelity, money. He took them all, listened to them with the stub of cigar going round and round, still gruff and impatient, but with a look in his eyes that clearly intimated a deep understanding, forgiving and nonjudgmental, a look of someone who could not be shocked, who had his own agonies and wasn't ashamed. When he heard enough he cut them off and told them whatever it was he had to offer. Sometimes he picked up a phone and in a very few words enlisted a medical specialist. Many times his counsel was no more complicated than: "Hey, Jimbo, you got to stop mewing and stand on your hind legs to her. Don't you think she expects that? Why else would she be workin' so hard at it?" Or he might simply listen and console, offering only the comfort of one who saw life in all perspectives at once, the pigeon droppings as well as the statue, and who could make others see it too. They almost always left feeling better, not infrequently laughing, glad to have found solace in someone so wise, so knowing, a man who also found humor in the leavings of incontinent wildlife.

Cassidy had been in the main training room the day Jolie Benson came in, a brilliant athlete from south Florida who could play very nearly any skill position on the football field; Jolie, who had in his junior year in high school walked into his father's study to find the old man in his leather chair, .38 in hand and a lap full of gristle that Jolie could never quite forget and which now reduced his voice to a moist stutter, a problem so debilitating at times he could not communicate at all.

Brady had been taping yet another anonymous ankle, muttering as usual to himself, when Jolie burst in and commenced with his routine: "Bray . . . Bray . . . Bray . . . Bray-dee, I . . . I . . . I . . ." Brady watched for a few seconds, fingering a roll of tape, his great sad eyes studying Jolie intently. Then finally he snapped: "Jolie! Cut it out! What the hell do you want?" And Jolie just jumped back in shock and suddenly started talking almost normally, telling Brady whatever it was he had come in to say. This was no screenwriter's permanent cure, of course, and Brady did not for a moment believe he could work such miracles. He knew the soul could sustain far deeper wounds than he could reach with his ultrasound machines, his muscle balm, ice packs, and gruff humanity. But Brady could, by God, get a man to talk straight to him, even one whose teenage eyes had beheld infinite sorrows; that was the way you talked to him. You weren't allowed to hide behind your own illusions because Brady did not hide behind his. It was little wonder that generations of athletes departed Southeastern with such a wry and honest love for Brady Grapehouse.

One day when Danny Ingram wandered into the main training room to get some tape for the track team, he saw Brady stalking briskly to the water fountain. Jolie Benson was sitting inside the glass enclosure, staring at the far wall, desolate tears falling unnoticed onto his incredible hands. Danny stopped his fiddling to ask Brady what was wrong and only then saw (he would swear) large tears also rolling down the round impish cheeks of the head trainer.

"What the hell do you want?" Brady croaked.

"Nothin', Brade," Danny mumbled, grabbing the tube of tape rolls and scrambling for the door.

Brady was not exactly transparent, but most people figured him out sooner or later.

IT SEEMED LIKE THE NATURAL THING to do after wandering aimlessly around the campus all afternoon, but by the time he got to the training room, it was three o'clock and the basketball team was straggling in for their taping. Cassidy was still in shock. How could they do this? He was a star. He was captain of his team. Like the death of a close friend, this was a shock his mind wouldn't accept.

Brady and two of his adoring student assistants were holding forth, working quickly, efficiently, tearing the white strips with quick little rips. Normally it would have been a boisterous time, but since they were again bitterly discussing Brady's imminent departure, there was only pious anger. Jim Quillain, a six-six starting forward who was generally unemotional and soft-spoken, demanded that someone come up with a plan to fight Brady's unjust dismissal. The others were in general agreement. Yeah, Brade, why don't you do something?

Cassidy, realizing he had hit the rush hour, leaned in the doorway and watched. Some of the players nodded or gave a little wave, but most were engrossed in the discussion.

Finally, Brady stopped and stepped back from the ankle he was working on, hands on hips, cold cigar stump going round and round.

"Hey," he said impatiently, "let me tell you birds something. I mean someday you're going to be leaving this place and you'll have to go out there into that big shooting gallery your own selves. And you're gonna find there's a big . . . *monster* waiting for you. You're gonna find wonderful little surprises like this waiting for you all the time. It ain't all gettin' patted on the ass and 'hey, nice game, Jimbo fella' and 'hey, you look so pretty in your jock, let us give you a free ride.' No siree. That ain't the way she goes at all. But if you want to spend all your time fretting and sputtering about it, then that's what you'll do. But you won't get a hell of a lot else done, dollars to doughnuts. You better pay attention to that, boys, 'cause it's the straight scooby-doo. Old Brady's gonna do all right, but there ain't no law says you ain't gonna get a royal screwing 'stead of a round of applause, so if you want to bellyache, you can bellyache, but you could put your efforts into somethin' a lot more productive, like sendin' Care packages to the Rockefellers or somethin'."

"But Brade, they promised you . . ." Quillain's young, sincere face clearly showed the strain of trying to deal with something so patently unjust he couldn't accept it. *No one promised you there would be universal justice, you know,* Cassidy thought.

"Promises," Brady scoffed, taking his cigar out. "With a basketful of promises and your right hand you could probably jerk off, Quillain. But then, you're a lefty, aren't you?" They all roared, even Quillain, though he colored quickly. It was Brady at his finest, even here in his own pot of stew, trying to give them something that would work, something that—no matter how hard to face—was at least real and useful as opposed to the embroidered half-baked platitudes peddled elsewhere on campus. The straight scooby-doo was all they carried in Brady's training room, whether a brisk pronouncement that you were out for the season or a simple observation that life is sometimes a bitch; and nothing, not even the demise of Brady's own reign, was going to change that.

Brady had seen Cassidy standing by the door and knew exactly why he was there. He had heard two assistant football coaches talking about it at the Farley training table. He hoped the miler would stay around until he was through with the basketball team, but as the group was laughing at his last remark, he saw Cassidy turn with a smile and leave. Then he heard him chuckling down the hall. Maybe he will come back, Brady thought, at least I hope he does. He's one of the foxes and I'd like to see him uncaught until he hits his stride.

When Cassidy got to the field house, Denton was already dressing. Some of the others were there early and they quickly gathered around his locker, all talking at once.

"All right, all right." He raised his hands, asking for room. "There's nothing we can do about it now, so let's just leave it. I gotta get my run in. But I appreciate it, guys, really. I do appreciate it." They went reluctantly back to their routines. *Gotta get my run in?* he thought.

Cecil, the equipment room man, hobbled over and started mumbling something about how equipment privileges were to be shut off that day and locker privileges at the end of the week.

"Cecil." Cassidy was exasperated. "What kind of equipment do you think a distance man needs? I get from you every day a fresh towel and a pair of shorts. I don't even trouble you for a jock, for chrissakes. And the shoes are mine, the gift of a generous manufacturer. I got a spare towel and shorts, though they aren't real clean. They can take their goddamn equipment and . . ." He took a deep breath, as Cecil stood there wide-eyed, staring up at the miler. It wasn't Cecil's fault, Cassidy knew, so he just waved his hand at the old man and smiled wearily. It was apology enough and Cecil limped sadly back to the equipment cage, back to his niche among the hanging gloves, the spiked and cleated shoes, the balls and bats, vaulting poles, racket-stringing post, busted hurdles; back to the brassy clean male smell of sweat-stained leather from generations of boys who had long since played their games in the spring sunshine.

Denton watched the whole thing silently, already dressed, arms crossed on his bare chest.

"Let's run," he said.

C

DENTON SELECTED, for some reason, an obnoxious in-town course. Zip-zip they eclipsed spatters of neon clutter that is franchised America. Krispy Kreme, WhataBurger, Pizza Hut, Pizza Inn, Pizza 'n Brew, Pic 'n' Save, Pic 'n Pay, Pic 'n Scratch; and close at hand, always, the noxious spewing fuming chrome-and-rust serpent of the roaring two-laned variety that is America at quittin' time. This country at times stinks in the nostrils of the runner, Cassidy thought.

They had already passed their cul-de-sac, their sliver of serenity in the middle of town, an old part of Kernsville, a taste of a slower, bygone era, a small park area known as the Duck Pond. As they passed, Chief City Engineer Homer Windenberry had ceremoniously given the signal to his foreman, who pulled the lever, and with an inch and a quarter of high-grade Type S-1 molten asphalt, paved over a mama and seven itty-bitty ducklings.

Make no mistake about it, Kernsville was on the go.

"I AM SPEAKING of countrified air," Denton was saying, "where the body is not rattled apart by the insane pounding of heel against concrete. I am speaking of connective tissue given a fair shot—"

"I don't want—"

"A change, basically, of pace is what I'm getting at . . ."

"I don't want to sound like a crybaby, but I honestly never thought those clowns would actually go so far as to—"

"Cut their own throats? Don't kid yourself, Cass, they don't give a flying you-know-what about spring sports, just so long as they're respectable. The pigskin is the only thing that cuts any ice down here in grit country. Do you know in Europe I get people coming up to me on the street? You think that kind of thing happens around here? No, Doobey may not be right, but this is his ballpark and he knows it."

"But old man Prigman—"

"Was the fire marshal on the *Hindenburg*."

Cassidy giggled.

"He and Doobey were joint lookouts at Pearl Harbor. Architects of the Walls of Jericho. Night watch on the *Titanic* . . ."

"Stop, I can't run." Cassidy was trying to run slightly bent over, making his little peacock noises. Finally he calmed down and they ran along in silence for a few moments.

"Rodent control officers during the Black Plague," said Denton, and they nearly had to stop altogether.

By the time they got back to the track Cassidy had not the slightest idea about what to do with his sorry life. But they had blown out the tubes on a 1:15 thirteen-miler and if the truth were known, he felt fine. Just fine.

23

More Horse Than Rider

THE SAME SCHEDULE that didn't allow much time for fretting about trivia likewise had no room for major catastrophes; Cassidy was content to follow the routine numbly. It was painful to no longer have a girl in his life, and soon he wouldn't have his teammates either.

Bruce Denton, who now saw himself as a man with a mission, came by to run *very* early. The varsity wasn't even moving around yet, so it was well short of 6:30 A.M.

The sun was nowhere near dawning and a thick fog was hung up in the rolling hills around Kernsville, turning it into a damp and quiet void inhabited by milkmen and sleepy policemen, where the whir and click of stoplights seemed inordinately loud in the chilled air. Soon Denton and Cassidy were outside the city limits, sliding quietly by acres of quiet pastures, occasionally leaving the fog below as they crested a hill. There was no sign of daylight yet and had they been less familiar with the course they would have had the impression they had already come a very long way, a notion that they suppressed neatly and automatically. Little tricks of the mind were important to them. They knew that it was psychologically easier to run a familiar course than a new one, so contrary to the advice in the magazines and jogger manuals, they seldom went exploring for changes of scenery. Because they were covering a good deal of ground at uniform, reasonably efficient traveling speeds, on any given training run they might run into and out of rainstorms, into or out of cities or counties, and into one geographically unique area and out of an altogether different one. To them the sensation was not unlike riding on some kind of very minimalist vehicle, one that traveled at a steady though unspectacular pace, and that would take them, they felt, just about anywhere they wanted to go. It was that feeling, perhaps, that inspired members of certain subspecies of their breed to embark on cross-continent excursions, hundred-mile trail runs, and other such madness.

Though the toil was arduous, they rarely spoke of the discomfort of training or racing in terms of pain; they knew that what gave pain its truly fearful dimension was a certain lack of familiarity. And these were sensations they knew very well.

That morning Denton was not talkative so Cassidy locked into a steady pace, allowing his mind to slip into the pleasant half-conscious neutral state that all runners develop; he was soon lost in the cool gray isolation of the fog.

The rumbling brought him out of it. He was tensing for the shock of big cold drops when he looked up and saw a herd of horses and ponies charging toward the fence in a pasture across from them. Denton said nothing.

The herd reached the fence, turned sharply to the right, and proceeded parallel to the runners at the same pace, looking straight ahead and running at a slow gallop with what appeared to be considerable pleasure. When they reached the corner of their pasture, they turned again and galloped off in a straight line directly away from the runners, disappearing as quickly as they had come. In a few seconds even the pounding of the hooves was gone.

Cassidy tottered. Could he have seen that?

"Was that an actual occurrence?" he asked.

"Damned if I know," said Denton.

"Do you suppose it was a coincidence?"

"Not a chance. Happens every time I run this course early. They always match my pace exactly. They were running with us."

"Riderless horses in the fog," Cassidy said mysteriously. "Do you suppose it's an omen of some kind?"

"Mountless riders in the mist," Denton said just as mysteriously. "That's what *we* are to them. Do you suppose we are omens?"

Cassidy sucked on his lower lip and said nothing. There are times, he thought, when you can't get away with *anything*.

DENTON DROVE OUT State Road 26 toward Newberry. It was a beautiful day, a crystal day with a shocking blue sky; a day for mock heroics and knowing smiles.

"I can't wait to hear the plan," Cassidy said.

"And I can't wait to tell you. Meanwhile, let's not look to horsies and moo-cows for auguries. Let us, as they say, keep our eye on the ball."

"Okay."

"And I have a little story to tell you"—he gave a little Uncle Remus kind of chuckle—"that I think you will find real entertaining." Cassidy clapped his hands stiffly, childlike.

"But first, I'd like to know some things. Like, has anyone around campus called to offer help of any kind?"

"Oh, sure, I guess so. Hosford said there have been calls from a bunch of student government honchos, Father Gannon at the Catholic Student Center, the ACLU guy in town, Feldman. And, of course, all the guys want to march, boycott, demonstrate, et cetera, et cetera. Hell, for all I know, they're getting up another petition."

"Well, at least they're on your side."

"Hell, *everyone* seems to be on my side. Even old Doobey said he was doing it for my own good. I get a few more people on my side and my side is going to sink."

Denton said nothing.

"And the worst is not even out yet. They have this statement—Prigman and Doobey—I mean, that they are releasing to the press this afternoon. It accuses certain spring sports athletes, of which I am singled out as the quote ringleader unquote, of fomenting a veritable rebellion among the various athletes and of infecting the football team with radical-type thinking. They claim this process has been going on right under their unsuspecting noses since the football season and they casually mention those close games with Tennessee and Auburn right there at the end of the season. Jesus!"

Denton rolled his window all the way down, letting the air blast in, forcing him to talk above the roar.

"Well, let me tell you my little story before you get all worked up. We had a black half-miler at my college in Ohio, a very talented kid who managed to run 1:47.5 as a junior. And that looked like he was just warming up. Beautiful runner. This kid was a writer also; took it seriously and all, and actually he wasn't too bad. I read some of his stuff in the school quarterly—don't give me that look; I know what you think of my literary judgment. Anyway, this guy had a story in the magazine that had the word 'fuck' in it. It wasn't a particularly dirty story. Matter of fact, it was about some athletes and the word was used in some locker-room dialogue. It wasn't even his best story. But anyway, the administration got a collective heart flutter; they confiscated all the issues of the thing right off the presses and fired everybody they could think of who didn't have their asses covered. As you can gather, our school was not exactly a bastion of libertarian thinking.

"Our 880 man was a whale of a celebrity," Denton continued. "A suit was filed and some federal judge informed the administration that as far as he knew the First Amendment was still on the books. It was a fine day for the good guys."

They rode in silence for a while. Cassidy turned to Denton. "And?"

"And the kid ran 1:56 that year and then disappeared altogether."

THE LITTLE A-FRAME CABIN was back up in a thicket of tall straight pines and waist-thick live oak and looked like it belonged. There were stacks of paneling and other wood lying around inside along with other signs of ongoing construction; the whole place had the clean, chewing-gum-sweet smell of cut wood. Cassidy kicked and poked around, trying to act like a man who knew his way around a construction site.

"It's great," Cassidy said, taking the mug of coffee Denton held out. "Whose is it?"

"It's mine."

"Yours?"

"Right. Come on over here and sit down where it's not so dusty. I guess this will be a day of revelations, in a manner of speaking, and I'm telling you right now, it's all in the strictest of confidence. Also, I don't want you to go drawing any conclusions or moralizing on me until you have heard me out."

"All right," Cassidy said. What next? he wondered.

"The place is mine, along with fifteen acres, lock, stock, and septic tank. I've had my brother-in-law working on it for nearly a year, but now he's gone back to school in Boston. We've done it all ourselves. It's still a little rough around the edges, but when I finish my doctorate, I plan to move Jeannie and myself out here and grow some of the goddamnedest exotic plants you have ever laid eyes on. There are two greenhouses in skeletal stages in the back right now . . ."

"Yes, but—"

"Let me tell you and then you can handle it any way you want to. This is partly about money, as you probably guessed. I don't know how much you know about this kind of thing, but here it is: I was paid $25,000 in cash to wear blank brand of track shoes in the Olympic 5000-meter final. I have no personal knowledge, but I suspect that everyone in that race had some kind of deal. Myself, I had a signed and witnessed contract that probably would have stood up in a court of law, though I would have never run again as an amateur if it had ever gone that far."

"They gave you $25,000 . . ."

"Cashier's check. Negotiated in a bank in Luxembourg."

"But what if—"

"*They* found out? *They* don't want to know. I suppose if they had their noses rubbed in it, they would go huffing and puffing around and start suspending people. But, if you haven't figured it out yet, the guys that run sports are lightweights; old jocks that didn't make it or couldn't leave it behind. They don't want any trouble, they just want their blazer patches and their freebie trips. And see, all the shoe contracts have a clause guaranteeing a legal defense against any attack on an athlete's amateur status caused by the payment. But like I say, the federations don't want to know about it. The communist-bloc countries have been supporting their athletes completely; the Europeans have blatantly been getting paid for years; even the American sprinters have been raking it in when they go over there. Only in the past few years have our distance runners been, uh, taken care of."

"Twenty-five *grand* . . ."

"Oh, that's not all, of course. There were bonus clauses built in for various highly unlikely potentialities, such as my winning the race or setting a world record. The amounts reflected the startling odds against me, of course, and big numbers are just so much fun for businessmen to throw around when they're just so many paper zeroes."

Denton looked at Cassidy, who seemed a little shocked.

"So, I don't want to bore you with the details, but to make a long story short, I find myself quite pleasantly, uh, *situated*. Remember, now, this is still in the strictest of confidence."

Cassidy nodded, solemn.

"And something else, Quenton, this is not to be considered the view from the top of the mountain either. I am not trying to get you pumped up for that great bonanza waiting behind door number three . . ."

"What *is* this to be considered, Bruce?"

"In the first place, I don't appreciate that tone. But I guess it is probably to be expected, at least until you get used to the idea. But let us just call this a modest proposal. I want you to understand a little bit of what it's all about out there, I suppose, before you go making any big decisions about your future. In a way, what has happened to you is a part of what it's like out there."

Denton stretched his legs out on a stack of paneling, leaned back against the wall, and gestured to Cassidy to make himself comfortable.

"I was pretty much like you at one time—and I'm going to do my best to avoid melodramatics here—I busted my hump for six years for a chance to stand on that platform and have some old fart in a blazer and straw hat put that medal around my neck. That's really all I was up to, Quenton. I wanted to stand up there and let a little tear roll down my cheek while they played the Mouseketeer Club song and the old glad rag climbed the pole. I wanted to look into the camera while old Howard interviewed me and say: Hey, Ma! Look at me! I'm the King Bee!"

"And?"

"And that's what I did. It was just great, Quenton, greatest experience of my life, no question about it. But then I found out that everything in the land of the free is not exactly free, but negotiable. Which doesn't mean much really, unless you let it."

"I'm not sure that I follow."

"Oh, it's an all-weather loony bin out there, Quenton, you know that. They're up to their assholes in fried chicken and nondairy creamer; they're running around selling each other life insurance and trading wives at Tupperware parties. Their children are slack-jawed and aspire to drive stereophonic vans, and everyone expects their stars—of whatever category—to be modest and well paid."

"I don't believe I am as naïve as—"

"And before they got around to finding out I *was* a star, I couldn't get myself a bus ticket to the Kansas Relays, much less make a fortune for running a race. Would you like to know how I got to the Drake Relays that first year when I ran that 27:22?"

"They didn't invite you?"

"Hell no, they didn't invite me. Cornwall called them and said he had a graduate runner doing twenty-eight minutes in time trials and they laughed and asked him did he time the guy with an alarm clock. So I called them back myself and asked if they would enter me if I got there on my own. They said sure. Good old American business, right? Never turn down the freebie. So I went out and borrowed enough from a small loan company for a one-way ticket. This is how your basic free enterprise system develops its Olympic champions of tomorrow."

"One way?"

"And Frank Shorter sent me an unused portion of a ticket he had from San Francisco to Atlanta; I had it changed and got back on that."

"Shorter did that? So you could go out and run against him?"

"Not for that. He just wanted me to have a chance. He had

been through the same thing himself. Right after he got out of Yale and was just bumming around, training and trying to get into meets, he lived on the floor of my dorm room. This was before Jeannie and I got married. Frank and I trained, slept, cooked on a hot plate, and dreamed about becoming stars. I tell you, I would have done well in that race if I had had to crawl across the finish line on my hands and knees. So that's it. Beforehand I had these people more or less laughing at me. But after that race, it was, oh Bruce this and gosh Bruce that. I told Shorter I couldn't believe it. He just laughed; he knew. He had been through it all himself."

"I recall a song about too many TV dinners, about how everyone loves a winner . . ."

Denton smiled. "You're getting the picture." He stood, stretched mightily, sat again.

"But more to the point," Denton said. "What I'm getting at is, I'm advising that you practice a certain amount of discretion. I am advising regrouping, getting some country air, thumping some soft trails . . ."

"Out here?" Cassidy looked around. "What about school, the athletic department thing. What about *girls,* for crying out—"

"The vertical smile? Well, the prospects are limited. Also graduate-level bull sessions, extended beer swilling, elaborate practical, uh, jokes of a legal nature. All limited."

"I see your point."

"For a long time I didn't believe you could make it, Quenton. I still don't know, really. You seemed to have almost too much going for you. It's a very intangible thing. A boxing champion from the ghetto expresses his anger and frustration with a lightning left cross. Other than that, he's inarticulate. You've never been at a loss for words, Quenton. And you've never seemed hungry enough, frankly."

Denton stood, walked back to the kitchen to refill his coffee mug.

"To be brutally honest with you, Quenton," he said, "I always figured that once you did four minutes, that would have been about it for you." He said this very quietly, almost sadly.

It was deadly quiet in the little house. Cassidy swallowed. Denton just looked at him, waiting for some kind of response. But all Cassidy could think was, *My God, you're right, you're right! How could I have not known?*

Finally, Cassidy said very softly: "I seem to have solved that problem. I don't exactly have anything going for me now. They've taken away—"

Denton slammed his mug down. "*They* have taken away *nothing*! *THEY* are irrelevant! That's what I want you to understand!"

"I must be slow or something . . ."

"Move out here, Quenton, and train. Train your guts out. Drop out of school, forget that mess for a while, it's nothing but trouble. They are all a bunch of small men with weak minds and tiny little goals for themselves; they'll cause you nothing but grief. There are great trails out here and a little grassy field for intervals. You can run barefoot on it the way you like to. It'd be ideal, a runner's paradise."

"Drop out of school?"

"You're a bright boy, you can do that diploma business anytime. But I've been watching you since last year, Quenton, watching you very closely. Ever since you ran that four flat—"

"Four flat point three."

"All right, four flat point three. I've been watching you, your training, the way you handled breakdowns, everything. I've been watching, Quenton, and I can tell you that physically you are getting close. Very close. Do you know what I mean?" He didn't wait for an answer, but strode to the big picture window that took up most of the front of the structure.

"People conceptualize conditioning in different ways," he said. "Some think it's a ladder straight up. Others see plateaus, blockages, ceilings. I see it as a geometric spiraling upward, with each spin of the circle taking you a different distance upward. Some spins may even take you *downward,* just gathering momentum for the next upswing. Sometimes you will work your fanny off and see very little gain; other times you will amaze yourself and not really know why. Training is training, it all seems to blend together after a while. What is going on inside is just a big puzzle. But my little spiral theory kind of gives it a perspective, don't you think?"

"Yes, but I don't see—"

"You've been in that momentum-gathering phase, Cass, is what I'm telling you. You've been in it for quite a while now and I think that—physically again—you're due. That four flat in San Diego was only the tip of the iceberg . . ."

"Four flat point one."

"All right, four flat point one. But your sights have been too low, Cass. You've always wanted to break four minutes so you could be a respected college miler. You wanted the other guys to look at you and say, hey, there goes Cassidy, the guy from Southeastern that runs four minutes."

"I'm not so sure that's such a—"

"Hell, forget about all that. *Go* for it, Quenton, is what I'm telling you, go for the big time, right now, at this precise point of your life, make up your mind to do it and do it. *Take your shot.*"

"But dropping out of school, Bruce. I'd feel like a quitter, like I was running away . . ."

For the second time this morning Cassidy thought Denton looked really irritated, impatient with him.

"Let me tell you something about winners and losers and quitters and other mythical fauna in these parts," Denton said. "That quarter-mile oval may be one of the few places in the world where the bastards can't screw you over, Quenton. That's because there's no place to hide out there. No way to fake it or charm your way through, no deals to be made. You know all about that stuff. You've talked about it. It's why you *became* a miler. The question now is whether you are prepared to live by it or whether it was just a bunch of words."

Quenton Cassidy thought about it a few moments, and then very quietly asked Denton exactly what his personal stake was in the whole affair.

"Let's say I am chronically attached to the underdog . . ."

"Bruce . . ."

"Let's say I am an ardent fan of that classical footrace, the mile run, that I have never had enough speed myself to—"

"Bruce . . ."

"Let's say I'm angling for a percentage of the take and—"

"Naw." Cassidy waved that off as well.

Denton sat beside Cassidy, removed his shoes and socks, and sat looking at his bony feet. Then he took a deep breath, and leaned over and pressed into the swollen skin of his bulbous red heels with his thumb. The surface remained indented, as if in modeling clay.

"They're full of lymph!"

"Yeah. They aren't as bad today as usual. Doc Stavius says the Achilles' sheath will become involved shortly and then it will be just a matter of time . . ."

"Bruce, I'm real sorry, I—"

"The hell with it. I would have liked another couple of seasons, I suppose, before hanging 'em up for good, but the hell with it. Connective tissue, Quenton, that's what gets everybody in the end. Pound around asphalt America long enough and you're going to wear something out for real. We can mold the muscles, you see . . ." He looked down at his knees sadly.

"We can strengthen the mind, temper the spirit, make the heart a goddamn turbine. But then a strand of gristle goes pop and presto you're a pedestrian."

"Can't they do anything?"

"Oh, you know how those things go. With a football player you can drill a hole in a bone and tie the goddamn things all over the place; but a distance runner gets so much as a stone bruise, he limps a thousand miles . . ."

"Bruce?"

"I'll probably hang around at meets . . ."

"Bruce?"

". . . wearing my old USA sweats, pretending to be warming up for a deuce or a 5000. What?"

"You tell me win one for the Gipper, I quit immediately."

24.
Moving Out

THERE WAS NOTHING SPECIAL about the room, but they say even a prisoner in the Bastille would wax sentimental over leaving his cell after languishing in it many years. Leaving the third floor of Doobey Hall filled Quenton Cassidy with both nostalgia and foreboding.

Mike Mobley came by and watched for a while, occupying nearly the whole door frame sadly as Cassidy puttered around with cardboard boxes and suitcases. Finally the weight man took a deep breath and held out his huge paw.

"Well, Captain Cassidy," he said. "I want you to know, I've always appreciated your . . . I mean, it's always been great the way you . . ." His big shoulders slumped wearily.

"Yes, indeed, Captain Mobley. I appreciate it, really I do. You take good care of that heaving arm, you hear?"

Mobley lumbered out shaking his head. Cassidy smiled. He would miss the harmless rituals. Soon others began dropping by and finally it got so distracting Cassidy closed the door and put up the little sign that said: THE KING IS NOT RECEIVING. No one really had anything to say anyway, they just sat around sighing and trying to make small talk.

When Cassidy had nearly finished packing, he sat down on a trunk and looked out the window at oak leaves that glistened with the dusty orange glow of sundown. But even as the room grew dim he did not bother to get up to switch on the light. Most of the others were soon downstairs at dinner, but he didn't feel like joining them. He took down his beloved posters. One showed Jim Ryun in agonizing full color running his world record mile at Bakersfield in 1966; another was a black-and-white blowup that Cassidy had had specially made, showing the classic moment in 1954 when Roger Bannister, his long hair flying straight against a gray August sky, passed John Landy as Landy looked to the inside to see how far back the Englishman might be, thereby losing in the final straight. I wonder how often Landy thinks about that moment, Cassidy mused. Maybe once a day?

The third poster had a sunflower on one side and a flowery message down the other: WAR IS HARMFUL TO CHILDREN AND OTHER LIVING THINGS. By asterisk it contained a typical Cassidy addendum: *Not to Mention Young Draft-Aged Males.

There was a slim profile shot of Kip Keino at full stride somewhere in his native Kenya, looking right into the camera and just grinning outrageously. Cassidy loved that one.

On the floor were various cardboard boxes and suitcases containing the effluvia of several years spent in a type of vortex; one box contained several fright wigs, a rubber chicken named Cletus, an Ella Fitzgerald mask, and a disappearing cane. A mesh bag held a diver's mask and snorkel, heavy jet fins, Hawaiian sling handle (the stainless steel shaft leaned in a corner), and several large conch shells with the hinges knocked out. There was a rolled-up WANTED DEAD OR ALIVE poster containing mug shots of the former president and attorney general of these United States; there was an eight-by-ten glossy of seer Jeane Dixon, a speaker on campus during his sophomore year, that contained in suspicious-looking handwriting the message: "Quenton, someday you will meet a tall, rich, and well-dressed stranger. He will put on a lab coat and replace your blood with embalming fluid. I practically guarantee it. Love, Jeane."

There was a cigar box full of cards, letters, and mementos of his time with Andrea, a box he did not have the gumption right now to go poking through. There was a brace of Frisbees and a collection of various-sized noses. One box held his record collection, which included *The Buttoned-Down Mind of Bob Newhart,* some early Shelley Berman, Mort Sahl, Vaughn Meader, et al. There was a sound-effects record offering exploding dynamite, grinding winches, breaking dishes, and assorted animals in varying stages of distress (a popular cut was the turkey section). There were antiwar crooners, and Kingston Trios gone cloudy with the scratches of time. A scrapbook was fat and sloppy with plane tickets, pages ripped out of meet programs, newspaper clippings. The photographs were mostly of Denton or some California sprinter or vaulter; Cassidy's appearances were generally in agate type. Though there were two large cardboard boxes filled with trophies, medals, and meet watches that did not run well, most of his race booty had been sent home. There were stacks of paperbacks by Vonnegut, Mailer, Roth, and the little-known Richard Stein. There was a collection of columns by one Ron Wiggins entitled *The X-Rated Hen Suit.* A shoe box held the entire output of Harry Crews in paper.

One suitcase contained practically nothing but T-shirts: DRAKE RELAYS, RUN FOR FUN, PUMA, SPEED KILLS, I'M WITH STUPID, and THIN POWER.

There were two large boxes full of track shoes of every description; there were Adidas Gazelles in varying stages of decomposition, Puma interval trainers, several pairs of Tiger's Cortez, one pair of indoor pin spikes, an old pair of long spikes still dark with petroleum jelly and the mud of Chicago, road racing flats, nylon mesh Tigers for the steeplechase (still brand-new), and beach hack-arounds with no real mileage left in them. He thought: I have measured out my life in worn-out rubber.

He sat for a long time studying a pair of Adidas 9.9s that he had worn winning the conference mile the year before. Denton had given them to him one day in the locker room. He had tossed them over casually and said: "You might like to have these, seeing as how we're the same size and all. But I want you to know these shoes have never been second." Then he had winked at Cassidy.

Three days later at the exact moment of truth, Cassidy had thrown up his fingers in the victory sign and made himself grin right at Denton, who was standing by the finish line. Not at all like himself, Denton had jumped in the air and whooped. The shoes still had not been second.

Cassidy sighed, tossed the 9.9s into the box with the others. They had all seen a lot, had their own decrepit personalities. He sighed again; the Trial of Miles, Miles of Trials. Sometimes it seemed sad to him and he really didn't know why.

A timid little tap at the door turned out mercifully to be Mizner, who was now living on campus. He plopped down on the bed and quietly helped observe the sentimentality of the moment. It finally made Cassidy nervous.

"How do you like civilian dorm life?" Cassidy asked.

"Three major water fights in four days if that tells you anything. I try to stay away as much as possible."

Cassidy nodded. He was sitting in his usual chair, feet propped up in the windowsill.

"Are you really going to do this hermit thing?" Mizner asked.

"I suppose. You know how we were always saying, what if a guy were to really shut everything out . . ."

"Yeah, well, when the nearest civilization is the town of New-berry, I don't think you have to worry about shutting out much of anything, except watermelon farmers, and I understand they're not all that rowdy. The question is, is this some kind of big push, for Pan Am, or maybe the, uh, Games?"

"Who the hell knows? It sounds silly to even talk about, doesn't it? You might as well say you're building a rocket ship to go to Mars but it won't be ready for a few years."

"And when it is, it may not fly."

"Right now I'm selecting the upholstery. Say, how have you been feeling anyway? Will they let you do anything yet?"

Mizner gave him chapter and verse of his medical situation. They talked on until it was nearly dark in the room and both of them began to realize it wasn't going to get any better. Mizner stood and held out his fine brown hand. Cassidy took it self-consciously.

"It has all turned out so differently," Mizner said. Cassidy lowered his eyes.

"Really something, isn't it? Last summer we were talking about going to Drake this year and how maybe we'd both try to learn to hurdle so we could run the steeple together, and then later in the summer for the hell of it we'd jump in a marathon somewhere . . ."

Mizner took a deep breath, slowly let it out. "I guess I'd bet-ter be going. Listen, you hang in there. And you better be tough next cross-country season because I believe we have some old business."

"I knew it! I knew Chicago really got to you, but you didn't let it show!"

"Nah," Mizner said, laughing. "Well, I guess I've had that coming for a long time. You don't know how many bad dreams

I've had about Quenton Cassidy being with me with a quarter to go." He shook his head, smiling sadly.

"Yeah, well . . ."

"Hey, listen, Quenton—I never call you that, do I?—anyway, Cass, there's something I want to say that I guess I wouldn't get around to except for a deal like this . . ."

"Hey, Mize, you don't need to . . ."

"Oh, yes I do. What I want to say is that, well, I know we joke around a lot, what with Bruce the way he is and all. But we both know that when you get right down to it, the guy is pretty damned intimidating. It's only because we *know* him that . . ." Mizner swallowed.

"And Cass, we've been friends for a long time now . . ." He lowered his head, as if too weary to go on. Cassidy looked out the window.

"Listen, Mize," he said.

"Quenton, you know how sometimes on a really bad one when you realize how it's going to be real early, like the second lap, and there's just nothing you can do about it except tuck in and gut it out? And how hard it is for the other two who are not running to sit and watch and know what is happening and not be able to do anything about it? Christ, Cass, I've seen you go through it so many times and every time just when I think it has finally gotten to you for once and you are going to slack off on yourself a little bit, you . . . just come blowing out of that last turn like some goddamn maniac and I just . . ." His voice cracked and he turned away slightly. Cassidy was distressed.

"Jerry, it's the same with you. You know how it's been. The same for all three of us. Bruce too."

"Yeah," Mizner said, "but with him there's no mystery left in it."

Cassidy considered that.

"Not as much," he admitted.

"And it's gotten so there's not much left with you either, Cass, is what I'm trying to say. I guess I've gotten so I'm not really afraid for you that much anymore."

Cassidy studied his bare feet. He never in his life expected to hear such a confession and he couldn't think of anything to say.

"Aw, who the hell knows?" Mizner laughed. "I just wanted you to know I've become kind of a fan, that's all. Hey, don't let it get to you out in the boonies. One of these days this mess will settle down and it will be just like it always was." He had almost closed the door when he stuck his head back in and gave Cassidy the old smile, white teeth flashing against the dark background of his face.

"Miles of Trials," he said.

"Yes." Cassidy smiled back. "Yes, indeed."

The door closed softly. Cassidy sat alone on the sheetless mattress in the eerie gloom, staring at the barren room which was even now growing cold to his mind. Finally he heard the horn of Denton's car down below. He exhaled deeply and stood up. Quenton Cassidy was a believer in all manner of Comebacks and Second Chances, but whatever happened, it would *not* be like it always was.

Never, ever again.

25.

The Woods

LIFE IN THE CABIN had an unusual effect on Cassidy. The runners had always leavened the unavoidable solitude of their sport with the social atmosphere of the team, but now that Cassidy's isolation was geographical as well as physical, he slipped toward goofiness. He read massively. When that didn't do it and his natural gregariousness boiled over, he began to carry on conversations with inanimate objects.

"Why do you do this to me?" he would ask of a broken shoelace.

"Getting a little grubby, aren't we?" he suggested to the coffeepot one morning.

These one-sided conversations had begun, naturally enough, during the first few days when he had tried watching television

(Denton brought a little portable, thinking the diversion might help).

"Oh, let's the fuck not!" he had cried to the silver-haired uncle type who had implored: "Let's talk for just a moment about constipation." And when the prim and proper lard ass Aunt Nell walked into the young bride's new house, turned up her little snout, and made a just barely overheard remark about "house-i-tosis," Cassidy got up from his chair, muttering softly: that, really, will not do. He unplugged the set, wrapped the cord around the handle, and placed it in the oven (which he used only for heating the kitchen).

"You're going to stay in there until you goddamn well learn some manners," he informed Aunt Nell, and then promptly forgot about her. And not just her. He also forgot about the legions of thrombosed bridge partners, impotent husbands, adorably precocious children, and finicky pets. Cassidy thought: *Descendants of spelling bee champions and fellers of giant trees are harangued about the slings and arrows of lower tract distress. A monk sets himself afire in the street and folks run for the marshmallows. Or am I being picky?*

After that, when he wasn't running or sleeping, he just read.

When his eyes tired, he tried just sitting.

He began to feel like the lama on a mountaintop who is so finely tuned he senses the very food moving through his body, the air molecules penetrating lung sacs and being dispersed to the far-flung cells. He treated such newfound sensitivity not with pride but suspicion; Eastern religious gimmickry was endorsed enthusiastically by any number of dorm-bound adolescents but Quenton Cassidy abjured the crowd.

He quickly settled into a mesmerizing pattern of hard training, reading, eating his simple fare, sleeping like a wintering bear, and talking to the pots and pans.

"I'm going nuts," he informed himself happily in the mirror one morning.

£

DENTON CAME OUT on weekends, and after training together they worked on the greenhouses in back. Once he had the idea, Cassidy was able to hammer away by himself during the week, but when the February rains started, he was deprived even of this activity for the most part.

Denton, however, was crafty, and understood all too well the logistics of single-minded effort. He often brought fresh reading material for the hermit, books that zeroed in on a subject of a mutual interest. Cassidy devoured them all: Sillitoe's *The Loneliness of the Long Distance Runner,* Roger Bannister's urbane *The Four-Minute Mile,* Peter Snell's *No Bugles, No Drums,* a novel called *The Olympian* by Brian Glanville (not bad at all), another called *The Games* by Hugh Atkinson (pretty awful). Soon Cassidy felt he had read everything ever written about running. He pored over Fred Wilt's *How They Train,* a compilation of the training schedules of the elite and near-elite. It was helpful to him, this little library, for it kept him focused on his task. The novels, while generally flawed technically in one way or another (sometimes tragically so), occasionally clumsily captured certain elements of his own striving; he found them comforting. The biographies were more esoteric, suffered no attempt at art, and delighted him no end. From them he learned he was not really alone. He especially loved *A Clean Pair of Heels,* the story of the great New Zealand distance man Murray Halberg.

Often the day after a late-night reading jag, he took to the country roads and wooded trails with renewed energy, comparing his impressions to his historical or fictional counterparts. He decided that no one had quite captured the strained satisfaction of tooling through the middle miles of a hard fifteen-mile run; but then he thought, some experiences do not easily lend themselves to descriptions by mere word butchers.

It was a good thing, he decided, not to have everything available in capsule form. Few others mentioned how wonderful, delicious, and life-giving it was just to *stop* sometimes, at the end of a run, with such a pitiful thirst (with swollen tongue and all) that the runner is convinced he knows what it would be like to die in the desert; when that first beer won't be like liquid at all but just a kind of wonderful fire burning down a viscous throat.

But all the books helped him in some way or another. Quenton Cassidy was not enthusiastically going about the heady business of breaking world records or capturing some coveted prize; such ideas would have been laughable to him in the bland grind of his daily routine. He was merely trying to slip into a lifestyle that he could live with, strenuous but not unendurable by any means, out of which, if the corpuscles and the capillaries and the electrolytes were properly aligned in their own mysterious configurations, he might do even better something that he had already done quite well.

He was trying to switch gears; at least that is how he thought of it. And though it was a somewhat frightful thing to contemplate for very long, he really *was* pulling out all the stops. After this he would have no excuses, ever again.

This here train, he thought, *she's boun' for glory*.

Ain't she?

26

Recon Work

FORAYS: he liked the sound of the word, implying as it did woodsy recon work. Illicit after-hours excitement for the young rogue about town. What the hell, he thought, I'm getting twenty-three blooming miles a day. Thus he found himself for the first time in Newberry's only bar, which was thankfully not called the Dew Drop Inn, being more or less alternately ignored and scowled at by any number of local good old boys who figured this bird was looking for trouble.

But then they also noticed that he looked a little on the, well, *wiry* side. They kept their distance.

The jukebox twanged away in the corner, evoking the bucolic muse. Cassidy picked up a napkin and began a soggy composition, a surefire country song sensation entitled: "Don't Send No Form Letter to Your Sweetheart After You Done Mass-mailed Your

Love All over Town." About halfway through, right after a line that said: "This is where the teardrops dry up for me, *buster* . . ." he tired of the theme, started a new one with more appeal perhaps for the short-term credit community called: "Go Put Your Love on Master Charge, You Got No Credit Line with Me."

Down at the end of the bar, an old-timer engaged the proprietor in a loud, showy mock-argument in order to demonstrate his status as a regular:

"Leroy, I swear if you don't cut this Wild Turkey . . ."

"Now, James Lee, I'll run you ass right on outa here . . ."

I am back in real life again, Cassidy thought, in the dank ambience of a Panhandle bar amid a group of drivers of real pickup trucks. And that barmaid has got herself a fairly decent chassis packed in them Levi's.

"Real pretty hair," he told her with what he still thought of as his impish grin, as she brought his third dizzy Pearl beer.

"You barkin' up the wrong sleeve, honey," she told him.

27

A Too Early Death

THE RAINS OF FEBRUARY CAME, bloating the pine forests and capturing all of life in the gray rumble of its clouds and the wetness of its seepage; all life except the unsmiling hermit who reluctantly left his dry nest in the same manner twice a day: standing on the small porch, savoring the last vestige of the eave's shelter, he surveyed the swollen clouds, the drenched colorless trees, the red mud seeping up through the pine needles like thin dirty blood, and with a sigh stepped gingerly into the first puddle like a cautious water bird. Then he struck out.

He had four pairs of training shoes, each of which remained wet all the time. If he could—by propping a pair up against the small electric heater—get them to a stage one might call "damp," he slipped them on with the greatest of pleasure. In some circles, there was some debate about training in spiked shoes. Cassidy rarely used them except to race in. They were thin on the bottom and afforded little protection to the heel and arch; he thought them risky. He had suffered in wet weather for years in shoes made of kangaroo leather and was grateful for the recent switch to nylon. But his thick-bottomed trainers still seemed to soak up a great deal of water; after a time he felt as if he were running with soggy pillows on his feet.

Some mornings he rose to find the huge mass of clouds rolled back, exposing a most brilliant, newly washed blue sky. He would pull on his slick shoes without a grumble and lope off along the soggy trail with his bounciest stride, wondering how he could have ever gotten himself into such a state. This, now *this,* he thought, was wonderful. All color and life had merely been disguised by a film of water. Birdies sang, moo-cows mooed, and Quenton Cassidy, a man with only the vaguest sort of plan, would sometimes laugh out loud in the middle of a run.

By the next afternoon, however, the clouds would have resumed their sentry and it would be pouring or sprinkling or at least threatening.

Such a winter, Cassidy thought bitterly, *is* always getting your hopes up. And he would resolve then to scowl through the next sunny day just by way of not being taken in. But it was a resolution quickly forgotten, such are the surges of a young heart given promise.

Were he completely honest with himself, he would have perhaps admitted that he didn't mind it so much, this rain that furnished the same kind of isolation as the dark of night. Snell used to say he didn't mind running in the rain because he always felt his opponents would have to be quite insane to be out in such weather, and while they were somewhere dry and cozy, he was gaining yet another few tenths of a second on them.

But occasionally at night Cassidy would sit over his training calendar and the full weight of it would descend on him as he stared at the figures. At those times he dared to wonder if it really was too much. He would think of the comradeship of Doobey Hall, the horseplay, the unpredictable silliness. His world now had too many sharp corners; he craved the soft contours of the feminine. Surely such longings were natural enough, he thought. Even the buffoonery of Jack Nubbins seemed a far-off entertainment taken too much for granted in happier times.

But out on the trails he slipped along in the soggy warm envelope of his own fierce body heat and needed precisely nothing. At these times, moving silently against the washed-out backdrop of countryside, his mind unfettered except for monitoring the steady six-minute pace, he went back to his childhood, back to the time of his too early death. He pondered what it meant, if anything; if anything at all.

Such a significant event as dying in childhood must take on some meaning in the end, he reasoned, if only a simple safety message, grade-school style: this is the Watch Bird saying look both ways before crossing the Santa Monica Freeway. But his death seemed to mean nothing.

On one of those rain-lashed afternoon runs, Cassidy finally decided that there was a great deal of vanity tied up in his demise, and in this respect perhaps Andrea had been right about his obsession. Perhaps it was *not* excellence he sought at all, but something else entirely. That part he would work on later. It had taken him a long time to arrive at the vanity part.

I used to frolic in the salt salt sea, he thought, and now my toes wrinkle white in this hillbilly mud.

WHEN HE WAS VERY YOUNG he had learned to slip into the sea and plummet like a stone to fifty, sixty feet, there to look around leisurely before floating back, calm and haughty in his control of the pale green waters. On rough, sunny days he would ride his bicycle across the Singer Island bridge and out to the inlet and scamper among the giant slippery boulders, at ease among the skittering crabs.

"What's he doing?" the white-kneed tourists would ask, seeing the waves crashing against jagged rocks so slick no one could even walk on them.

"Where are his parents? He'll be drowned!"

The child would spit into his mask, lean over and rinse it out in the sea, then grip the spear and wait for the right wave to come bashing frothily among the deadly crags and barnacles. Then, like a spirit, he would slip easily into the receding swell and, with a shiver, be gone.

Below, in the sudden quiet, he felt at once peaceful and serene in a terrain he knew better than his own room. The formation of rocks below was home for a school of big red snapper, skittish and crafty, which might let you get off one shot from a distance before disappearing for the day. At the cable crossing there would be sheepshead (easy marks—he ignored them) and schoolmaster snapper. Out toward the tip, closer to the open ocean, the real ocean, one could find just about anything; some days the sea would be literally alive. Quenton Cassidy had cavorted there like a young seal, sometimes actually feeling an illogical resentment at his addiction to air, a dependence that forced him regularly to make his way wanly to the top where he endured the noise and neon of an altogether different world.

The fishermen, wrinkled cigar-chomping retirees, cursed him for "scaring the fish" as they dangled their silly bait randomly in the sea. He felt the hunter's ancient disdain for the trapper. They almost never knew where he was.

The other kids were fascinated; they knew the waters too, but only he was known to go places they would never try, and bring back a handful of sand, a rusty nail, a little lump of coral and show them, laughing, the simple evidence of his prowess. Quenton Cassidy at ten already had his lungs.

The others wanted to know the secret. "Vitamin Z," he told them, laughing.

One time, though, his best friend had pleaded until, when they were alone on the end of the jetty late one afternoon, Cassidy told him: "You've got to make yourself calm, right down to the little blood veins in your fingertips, and when you are as calm as you can make yourself, then you make yourself like a rock and start sinking, and the most important thing is that you've got to not care. That's the hard part, the not-caring part. And the deeper you go and the colder it gets the more you have got to not care. And then when you start back up, back toward real life . . . then you've got to start caring again. A *lot*."

His father had a twenty-two-foot open fisherman that they took to the islands every summer and it was Quenton's job to fetch the anchor when it got stuck, silent and unmoving, on some ramp or drop-off far below.

"Now, Quentie, it's deep, you'd best put on a tank this time," the old man would say. The old man wore a pipe. He worked in photoengraving at the newspaper.

"It's okay, Pop." This as he flipped out of the boat with his mask and snorkel. If his heart raced with excitement of the challenge he would have to make it slow again, like he always did, calming himself, making himself into a rock and then slipping, slowly at first, then more rapidly as he went along, down into the darkening green, down to the cold depths where all the mysteries were. When he reached the bottom he would quickly work the anchor loose, then plant his feet in the sand and shoot upward, streaming bubbles all the way, wondering if he would make it this time.

One time he didn't make it and died there in the cool green waters.

There was a man from another boat on this trip, a lawyer his father knew and a good diver who had a grouper speared and holed up about forty feet down. The fellow was too tired to go back down and pull him out.

"Hey, Mr. C," he had called, "shame to waste those fillets. Whyn't you send that boy of yours down for a try?"

They had all heard as much as they wanted to about this little twerp, this little Quentie-fish and there was a distinct challenge in the invitation. His father looked at him resting there on the front platform and said: "Now, Quenton, you're very tired. You've been up and down in thirty feet all day long so if you don't feel like doing it, you don't have to."

But he was poking around for his gear already; the idea of leaving a dying fish tucked up under a coral head to suffer for days nearly made him weep. And he had always made it before no matter how bad it seemed, and the worse it seemed the sweeter the air was at the top when he finally broke through and got at it.

As he floated on the top, though, looking down to the coral head miniaturized below, he absentmindedly hyperventilated, thinking how far down it was, how tired he had become; by the time he took his last big gulp of air his system was all oxygen.

He was still peering around under the coral head and taking his time when he realized something was wrong. But by then it was too late; he just barely managed to trip the spring buckle on his weight belt and let the seven pounds of lead fall to the sandy bottom as he streaked toward the top. He was still twenty feet under when the blackness thundered in.

The limp body floated serenely to the top, and there bobbed gaily in the wind chop, looking for all the world like a lazy snorkeler, tracking his game. It took awhile before the elder Cassidy noticed how remarkably corpselike little Quenton looked, before he noticed the absence of any motion whatsoever; no little flips for forward motion, no play of the hands to turn or stop.

He was saying Jesus Jesus Jesus as he slashed the anchor rope with the fillet knife (and cut his own thumb down to white bone at the same time) and then roared over to pull the little gray body from the water, draining seawater from every orifice. There was seaweed in his teeth.

It was too much for the old man, it was too final-looking. The bottom of the boat was becoming slick with his own blood as he slid down onto the deck mumbling. But the others were more efficient. They had seen drownings before and were not so overcome with grief. They began blowing into the fouled little mouth and crushing the rib cage with strong hands. After half an hour there was some vomiting. He vomited and then they vomited. But color was coming back, and there was a faint pulse; finally some wild thrashing.

He had been floating around on the top for perhaps ten minutes, possibly more, and they had not held out a great deal of hope even as they frantically worked over him.

Then as he started coming back, although no one said anything, the big fear was that they were rejuvenating a mindless blob that would henceforth sit in some white-walled institution and drool contentedly.

But they did not know, could not know that the cardiovascular system they were priming with their frenzied efforts was capable of withstanding even greater shocks than it had that day. The lungs, the veins and vessels, the resilient throbbing heart; he had them all, even back then.

The next day they flew him back across the deep purple Gulf Stream at an altitude of one hundred feet; his blood was still so blue they feared to go higher. When he awoke finally in Good Samaritan Hospital in West Palm Beach he wanted to know what had happened to him. His father told him the story again. But every time Quenton went to sleep, he would forget it completely.

"Don't you remember, son? Don't you remember diving and . . ."

"I remember one time. I remember this day I was in the inlet working my way along the rocks at about thirty feet. And this little bull shark about four feet long was coming in from the real ocean; he was right in my path but I didn't move over, just kept swimming straight ahead. When he saw me he acted like he didn't care but he moved over a little to let me pass by. I was so ferocious with my sling, Dad, I wasn't afraid. I laughed because he was going so far in and I knew the hunting was better out near the tip."

Then he held his father, grabbed him and buried his head in the old man's chest and cried. His father had not seen him do anything like that for a long time.

This one, he thought, what is it with this one?

Nearly ten years later a land-bound Quenton Cassidy flew along on the soggy February trails and wondered the same thing.

28

Time . . .

O UTSIDE THE AFTERNOON RAINED ON.
    Cassidy leaned forward and placed all four legs of his chair on the floor carefully. He sighed heavily. The books were stacked up all around, finished and bleak-looking. He was tired of reading. He set his mug down on the table with a grunt. He was tired of tea.

He hauled himself to his feet, walked stiffly over to the picture window, a fogged square of chilled gray. He was tired of walking around with his joints creaking like an old man. He had a sudden passing desire for broccoli.

Afternoon workout was an hour and a half away; time to begin thinking about it. He was tired of psyching himself for workouts.

He was tired of being tired.

In reverse mirror script he wrote on the pane of cold glass: HELP! IMPRISONED IN FEBRUARY.

Little drops of excess moisture cried down from his letters as he looked out through them and waited for time to pass.

He stared out for a long time . . .

29

Twenty-four in the Rain

IT HAD NOT BEEN so awfully hard on Andrea Cleland, as she was beginning to tell herself lately. She had ended a few difficult relationships in the past but she was a very mature young lady and she managed. It was her maturity in fact that probably caused some of the distress. She was often a little too far ahead of the game to really take it seriously; though she had believed herself in love several times, it did not take her long to assay the true metal of the relationship. Before Cassidy she had begun to have some confidence in her ability to judge that most complex and shifty element in human dealings: motive.

It was not as if she had not had experience with ambitious men (or more accurately, ambitious boys); she knew very well when she was being sized up as a future charming hostess by the president of some fraternity, some bright, good-looking fellow who was easy to like and whose father owned an office supply outfit in Orlando. She chafed a little, but played the role. It was her sensitivity that made her more mature, gave her an edge over her hapless pursuers, and allowed her to set the boundaries. When it was over, she knew it first. And though she might grieve truly, it was a bittersweet emotion because though sorry, she was always sure of herself. She played hearts like fiddles.

And now this had to happen. She realized finally that she had never really understood Quenton Cassidy very well, that she had tried to use her past experience to take his measure and it didn't work. "His *cir*cuitry is all different," she told her twin sister. His ambition differed in essence as well as degree. Whereas with others she could tell the point at which she might assert certain proprietary rights (the very first hints of nesting behavior), with this runner there was never any question about her rearranging his priorities. This rankled her from the start. She might have the ability to make him miserable, perhaps, but she swayed him not an inch from his path. He told her as much, and she found out quickly he meant it. There was something in the ferocity of his dedication that challenged the formula of her femininity. She responded to the challenge without even realizing she was doing so.

To Quenton Cassidy, who knew little about women in general and less about Andrea in particular, their meandering, halfhearted breakup was a thing without reason. It would not abate with discussion, not be cured by soul-searching, not be resolved by agreement. They both recognized certain deep feelings that couldn't be denied, so why, Cassidy asked again and again, all these problems? She found it impossible to tell him that this simply wasn't the way she had imagined it would be. She was not experienced enough to know that it rarely is.

Cassidy thought that it was entirely fitting that all the underpinnings of his world should collapse at one time. When he took to the woods and his first nearly total solitude, it was almost with relief. At first it was.

THE HUGE OAK in front of Andrea's sorority house was over three hundred years old, had been an arm's thickness when Seminole Indians camped in the spot where the sorority house now stood, had shaded weary Spanish cowboys who kept herds on Payne's Prairie not five miles from there. This was at a time when a muddy, mosquito-infested fort named St. Augustine was a fledgling mission.

Now this old tree kept the steady rain off Quenton Cassidy, standing there in the night, heat-mist rising from his body, feeling anything but historic. He loved this old tree, and as he leaned against the incredibly gnarled trunk he thought: What does this old fellow care about it all? The strength of the ancient tree somehow soothed his misery.

The body heat from his run would keep him warm for a while longer, then he would start to get chilled and have to get moving again to stay warm. His bright nylon shorts and yellow T-shirt hung on him like colorful mud. He was drenched clear through to his childhood. At last he saw them drive up. They were laughing about something as they shared an umbrella to the porch. When the guy kissed her, Cassidy felt a stab of pain that was close to physical, and therefore within the penumbra of hurts he told himself he could bear. As she turned to go inside, Cassidy called to her. The fellow, peering out from under his umbrella, stopped halfway down the sidewalk and squinted toward Cassidy in the shadows of the old tree. The umbrella man looked grim. It appeared his duty was not yet finished; at first unsure of himself, he finally opted to return to the porch. Cassidy stepped out of the gloom and the porch light fell on him, gleaming in the rain. He called again.

"Quenton!" She was afraid she sounded a little too excited to see him. Then she remembered umbrella man, who was still coming. "It's all right, George. I'll see you Saturday." Still looking grim, he stalked back to his car and drove off. He had seen the way she ran out there in the rain like that, up to that crazy galoot in the gym shorts, who was *supposed* to be out of the picture.

"Cass, what in the world are you doing?" She gestured in a general manner, taking in the rain, the night, the silliness of it all. She seemed amused.

"Thought I would come to see you."

"But you're drenched. You've been standing—"

"I saw your light wasn't on, so I decided to wait for a while."

She tilted her head in amusement, like she used to do all the time, and finally put her arms around him. He seemed not to know what to do. She was getting drenched now too, but seemed not to notice.

She thought: He's harder now, even than before, all cartilage and bone and skin. She wondered if he was eating right; perhaps he would make himself sick. Something moved deep inside her and she had to stifle it willfully.

"I, uh, guess I was missing you," he said with his chin on her wet forehead, "and I suppose I got sick and tired of it all and just bolted on in here . . ." Something occurred to her and she leaned back away from him.

"You ran here!" It sounded like an accusation. He was puzzled.

"Yeah, I—"

"You ran into town from out there, twelve miles. And it's been raining like crazy all—"

"I don't have a car out there and—"

"Cass, you ran twelve miles in the rain to get here and you're going to have to run twelve miles back unless you call a cab or something . . ." He appeared unconcerned.

"It's my overdistance day anyway. Listen, Andrea, I wanted to talk to you because . . . are you listening?" She was shaking her head.

"Yes," she said softly.

"The last time we seemed to be like strangers. I've been feeling so horrible about the whole thing, I just get so frustrated that we can't seem to get anything straight . . ."

"Cass, I thought we had been all through that."

"I just keep thinking there must be some way to put it, some way that would allow you to understand."

"I think I understand." She looked into his eyes and thought that though once they seemed to balance the hardness of the rest of him, now they added to it.

"I think I've always understood," she said. "I just don't think I can live with it. Sometimes it seems too much for you too." He looked down, shook the rain from his forehead. She was nearly drenched now too.

"Don't you want to come in?" she asked.

"No. I'll be going, I guess. I'm starting to get chilled."

"Cass," she said, pulling him to her again. "What is this all going to get you? You've dropped out of school, you're not going to graduate with your class, you—"

"I ran a 3:58.6 mile the other night."

"What?"

"No race or anything. Just Bruce out there with a stopwatch and me, at ten o'clock at night. I had to go around the joggers even. Funny, I always dreamed how it would be going under four the first time, lining up, the pace, how the crowd would get excited when we came through the three quarters under three minutes . . ." He looked at her with a sad little smile. "But there it was, just me and Bruce—and a bunch of joggers wondering what in the hell was going on. Just another goddamn workout . . ." There was something that sounded vaguely like satisfaction in his voice.

"Quenton, why don't you come back into town? Where does it say you have to live like this, make yourself miserable like this?"

"It will all be over soon anyway. I'll be running Walton next month."

"And then what? You've already said you can't win. Even your exalted Bruce Denton says that. So then what do you do? Go back to your little cave and keep driving yourself until you are the one they talk about, the one they are afraid of? Is that what's important to you? Or maybe you'd be content to just go crazy trying? Then no one could say you compromised, could they? If something inside you just snapped?"

He looked down. She knew then he would not fight with her.

Then she did something that was not quite her and that did not work very well. It was a mistake and she knew it right away but it was such a precisely feminine gesture that it was perhaps dictated by some ancient genetic pattern she was helpless to control. With a pained little toss of the head she wrenched free and ran toward the porch; it was one of those shabby you'd-better-come-after-me-now gestures and she knew by the time she got to the porch that it was a bad show all the way around.

She turned to call, to try to take it back, perhaps.

But the runner had disappeared in the darkening rain.

30

Whirlpool

MARY LOU HUNSINGER sat in the gurgling whirlpool, checking her eyeliner in a small mirror; outside it still rained like a bitch. At that very moment somewhere out in the glistening night, a homeward-bound Quenton Cassidy came upon, was startled by, and hopped over a poor black snake trying to keep from drowning by crawling up to the high ground represented by State Road 26. Cassidy was just about halfway home.

Mary Lou's frown, of late an almost permanent fixture on her otherwise attractive face, was now a pouty badge of impatience at Dick Doobey, whom she thought rather a clod. On the home front her mother would be getting dinner for her two slope-headed sons, which meant that by the time she finally arrived, they would be as mean as a pack of starving blue jays (Mary Lou knew very well that as evil as the boys were, her mother was a shrew in her own right; she didn't even mean well).

She considered these bubbly interludes more or less in the line of duty. Not that she didn't take some basic carnal pleasure in them, but they required massive revetting of her expensively maintained hairdo. For all of its architectural integrity her bee-hive tended to sag in this steamy sanctum in much the same way as Mary Lou's own flagging hopes.

In this surreal chamber he brought her all manner of world-weariness, from his cold, church-crazed wife to the latest technical esoterica of his chosen profession. She bore it all with goodwill and no small effort to comfort and counsel. But what, after all, was she supposed to know about the weakside line-backer's responsibility in defensing the quarterback option out of the wishbone? As to the other, she had no difficulty whatever in flatly recommending that Doobey drop his "dry-hole little bitch" in order to take up with Mary Lou herself in some kind of more widely sanctioned arrangement. It was a scenario she had come to think of as the only nonfelonious way she would ever get out from under those killing monthly payments to five trust-ing department stores, two "friendly" small loan companies, and "the Master Charge," all of which her former mate—a two-fisted, bourbon-crazed paint and body man—had been so thoughtless as to leave as his only enduring legacy.

"Paint and body men's like a nationwide brotherhood, hon," he would warn ominously. "I could be in Tucson on Wednesday pulling down a hunnert and fifty dollars a day like that!" He would snap his stained fingers cockily. "Like doctors," he would say. "Always in demand." When he finally did take off, he had sense enough not to go to Tucson.

The powdery pink flamingo on the front lawn now seemed a mocking reminder of more opulent days when she had nothing better to do than to hop in the station wagon and go shoppin' to her heart's content. She never looked at the sun-faded little plaster bird standing forlornly on its rusting pipestem leg without wondering where it was exactly she had gone so wrong. They never mentioned this in Home Ec.

Wrestling with the viscous mathematical intricacies of 18 percent per annum interest, compounded monthly in accordance with federal statutes, she was driven first to secretarial work (she hated waitressing) and thence to Dick Doobey's private whirlpool.

The head coach finally arrived and let himself in with his own key. The strain of his staff meeting was still on his face. He apologized with the profuse sincerity of a man unquestionably willing to debase himself in order to maintain a good thing.

"That's all right, honey," she said. "I got nothin' better to do but sit here and get my little love button parboiled."

A flash of uncomplicated lust shot through Dick Doobey's loins as she giggled at her own line. Doobey noticed that she had brought a quart bottle of Southern Comfort, which now sat on the moist floor beside an open can of ginger ale. He made a grimace.

She watched him undress with contained distaste. He had long ago lost the trimness that was a by-product of his athletic days; his arms and neck were unattractively sunburned to the edges of his short-sleeved shirt, much in the manner of a gas station attendant.

His stomach rolled around loosely, the result of his long afternoons on the high pyramidal coaching tower, looking stern while drinking Budweiser (hidden in a Styrofoam Gatorade holder!), ostensibly surveying his minions scattered about the twenty-five-acre practice fields—a general watching his field commanders through powerful binoculars—but in actuality keeping a rather dutiful eye on Simmons Hall, the nursing school dormitory, where one could (were one extremely diligent) catch an occasional flash of nubile young breast or mouthwatering young thigh.

Dick Doobey loved his work.

He simply couldn't understand why some critics would wish to cause him anguish by suggesting that he was not doing a good job and should go away. He sincerely suspected communist influence of some kind.

When he had finally shed his damp garments and was settling his white bottom slowly into the scalding water opposite Mary Lou, he had managed to put out of his mind the distress of his latest staff meeting, where he had unhappily discovered once more that his staff was almost as much in the dark as he was. Football was becoming a damned complicated game and Doobey figured there was probably some foreign influence behind that as well. Some people were suggesting that they get soccer players to kick field goals. It was madness.

"How did it go, hon?" she asked, shifting around to allow room for his considerable bulk. He was almost settled now, leaning back and heaving a sigh of relief.

"Aw shit, honey, I don't know. I wanted that stumpfucker Erickson to read up some on this new wishbone formation—'member the one I tole you about where they can shift from weakside to strongside and run a option off the . . . no? Honey, I *just* tole you about it last week."

"Well, goddamn, angel, you know I don't remember that kinda stuff very well."

"Oh, well, it don't matter anyway," he said, sinking now to his neck in the roiling water. "I'll just have to do it myself, like everything else." He smiled at that, and began probing for her with his big toe.

"Now, honey, don't you want a drink or somethin'?" she asked.

"Of that sweet horse piss?" He continued probing. She dodged with precision, as her sex learns to do at an early age in the republic. A thought struck her.

"Hon, I finished typing that talk for tomorrow, it's on your desk if you want to take it home tonight."

"Christamighty. I forgot about that altogether." The misery he had almost shed now settled on him again and Mary Lou was sorry she had said anything.

"I wish I had some way to get outa that thing," he said mournfully.

"Why do you have to do it?"

"Old Man Prigman, uh, required it. Told me I'd never make conductor until I could face my own music. But Lord, standing up there in the plaza while a bunch of them snippy long-haired twats ask a bunch of asshole questions. Most of 'em *don't even go to football games!*"

"I thought that stuff was over."

"Over, hell. They still got that whatever they call it, Conscription of Athletes or whatever the hell they call themselves. Prigman said there wasn't a goddamn thing we could do about it except ignore it. Can you beat that? Here in America, and you can't do anything about people getting together to bad-mouth football!"

"Why can't you get rid of 'em?"

"Prigman said if we didn't nip it in the bud with that damn track guy, we would have to learn to live with it. Said we couldn't start throwing all of 'em out, it'd look too bad in the press. But boy, if I was runnin' the show . . ."

He rubbed his hands over his bristly head as if in some deep pain. "They keep issuing these mother-lovin' press releases. Jeezus!"

"Aw, honey," she said, taking his left foot, massaging gently. Slowly she worked her way up the hairy calf.

"There's gotta be something to do. I cain't keep up with all this stuff and operate a goddamn ass-kicking football team at the same time. That's more'n a full-time job by itself! More'n full-time!"

"Now, come on, honey," she said softly, still working upward. "We don't have to talk about that stuff all evenin', do we? Let's talk about somethin' else." Dick Doobey loosened with a moan under the onslaught of her simple ministrations. The toe probed feverishly.

"What do you want to do, hon?" he murmured softly.

"What do *you* want to do, angel?" she cooed back, as he began sinking lower and lower until finally his mouth was almost awash in the swirling water.

"Play alligator." He smiled evilly as his hot beady eyes slowly disappeared beneath the surface.

31

Irish Highs

W HEN NO ONE ANSWERED his knock, Bruce Denton wiped his muddy feet on the filthy welcome mat and went into the cabin. He was accustomed to the disarray, but surprised to see a bottle of Bushmills Irish whiskey open on the big cable spool that served as a kitchen table. He walked over, placed the cap back on the bottle, and picked up the book lying beside it; it was a softcover copy of *In Our Time*. He smiled.

"Hey, Nick," he called. "You in here, Nick?"

"Very funny," Quenton Cassidy croaked from behind a stack of paneling. He lay just under the front window, parallel to it, almost completely obscured by the lumber. Denton walked over and sat down on the stack of wood. Cassidy smiled up at him, a coffee mug rising and falling on his chest (it contained several

nearly melted ice cubes and probably no coffee, Denton sur-
mised).

"So . . ." Denton let the word hang.

"I thought you were coming out here yesterday, jerk," Cassidy
said pleasantly.

"Ah yes, well, sorry about that. Jeannie got to feeling bad and
I ran her by the infirmary. We are, uh, waiting for word on the
rabbit or whatever it is they do these days. When I got back it
was dark, so I decided to come today."

"Oh. Pitter-patter of little spikes around the house . . ." Cassidy yawned, did not appear very interested.

"So. What's the occasion? Or am I being too personal?"

"Occasion? Since when does a fellow have to have an occasion
to bend an elbow?" Cassidy asked. Denton knew that Cassidy
drank a lot of beer, but had never seen him take anything harder.
He was partially amused, partially alarmed, but only the amusement showed.

"Doing a little reading, eh? What's this?" He picked up the
paperback folded open beside Cassidy and turned it over to look
at the cover.

It showed a young man sitting on a bench in a locker room
putting on Tiger training flats; behind him an older man stood,
towel around his waist as if he were about to yank it off with a
cry of *Lookee here!* Cassidy giggled at him.

"That, my friend, is a book that explores a much overlooked
and steadily growing athletic minority, the homosexual distance
runner."

"Oh yeah?" Denton was leafing through the book. "What's
the main . . . I mean, what do they, uh, you know . . . *do?*"

"I can see, sir, that you are a man of little sophistication.
These fellows train themselves to a fine edge while maintaining
dalliances with their ex-marine coaches, they fatten themselves
up on yogurt and walnuts, and then they go out and run fantastic
races despite the overwhelming social pressures brought to bear.

Oh yes, they also 'rip off' fifty-seven-second quarters in morning workouts. But mostly . . ." He got up on his elbows so he could look Denton in the eyes. "Mostly they kind of lay around the locker room admiring each other's tawny hamstrings." He giggled again.

"Hmmm. Is this some latent prejudice of yours finally making its way out of the closet? I thought you were one of those put-it-into-whatever-you-want-or-whoever-you-want kind of fellows."

"Look, my view of sexual matters is that consenting adults should be allowed to run over each other with hay balers, if that's their fondest desire. So long, of course, as they don't do it in front of the children. Or lovers of harvesting equipment."

Denton nodded, but he seemed engrossed in a passage in the book. His forehead wrinkled as he read for a few moments. Finally he tossed the book back on the floor.

"Whew!" he said.

"See what I mean? Now really, what does how you get your jollies have to do with anything? So what if I'm out here whipping my wire fifteen times a day? Who cares?"

"Yes, well, I see you're a little overwrought about this . . ."

"Overwrought, hell. I'm drunk as a skunk." He giggled again. "I'm so fine-tuned I get blipped from a tumbler of Dr Pepper."

Denton couldn't help laughing. "How about the Hem's Michigan stories I brought?" he gestured back toward the table.

"Yes, I liked them pretty much. Except for all the stiff-upper-lip crap. But the guy went out and did things, you know; I mean you could tell he really did those things, *knew* about them before going out and shooting his mouth off. He just sat down and tried to tell it as honestly as he could. That's a shitload better than sitting around New York with a bunch of other artistes diddling each other and writing about the state of being Jewish, or how anguishing it is to be an anguished writer. But then again . . ." His elbows were tiring, he flattened out on the floor again.

"Who cares?"

". . . who cares indeed?" Cassidy sighed. Denton thought: here is a man who's been alone too long.

"Christ, Bruce, I've got to get out of this hole. Take me to some food, to a place with people I can snarl at, waitresses in panty hose, a place with that hallmark of civilization, a salad bar with fake bacon bits . . ."

"Just what I had in mind, assuming you can walk. Steady there," Denton said. Cassidy was struggling stiffly to his feet.

"Did you run today?" Denton asked, helping him up.

"Can a fish tread water? Hell yes, I ran today. You think I'm out here to taunt the farmers? I'm going to take a shower."

Denton saw the training calendar on the floor where Cassidy had been lying. He picked it up and studied it for a moment, finally letting out a low whistle.

"What in the hell were you doing running thirty-four goddamn miles yesterday? Are you going bonkers or what?"

Cassidy stuck his head out of the bathroom. "I ran into town last night. See, I thought my good friend and coach was going to be coming out to do a workout with me and he didn't show up, see? Oh hell. I went in to see Andrea. It was a mistake . . ."

"Okay. Fair enough. I won't stand you up anymore. I know this is rough out here sometimes, but I thought the Andrea business was all over with, wasn't it?"

But the bathroom door was closed. In the shower Cassidy crooned off-key: *"an' all of us here are just more than contented . . . to be livin' and dyin' in three-quarter time . . ."*

Cassidy was still in a good mood as they drove into town. Denton switched on the windshield wipers as they hit a mild shower. The intensity of the rains had waned lately.

"Now, if you'll settle back," Denton said, "I'll give you a rundown on the news. It's short, and not very pleasant."

Denton began telling Cassidy about the organization formed by campus athletes called Coalition of Southeastern University Athletes.

Its express purpose was talking, negotiating, and otherwise "dealing" with the Athletic Association, Denton told him. When the group announced its formation, the media blitz that had so disrupted Dick Doobey's life at the time of the Awesome Midnight Raid returned with a vengeance. Sportswriters rankled at the idea of an athlete's "union" and wanted to know how conditions could be so bad as to necessitate collective bargaining in jockdom. No one, least of all Dick Doobey, was able to provide a satisfactory answer. The athletes simply told reporters that as the writers did not live in the regime, they could hardly understand the Zeitgeist. More meetings were held, statements were released, Quenton Cassidy (who had apparently disappeared altogether) was eulogized as a martyred saint or damned as a self-serving rabble-rouser. There had been editorial comment on some sports pages, Denton told Cassidy, "that would boggle your noodle." A progressive commentator at the *Pensacola News Journal* suggested capital punishment for ungrateful student athletes.

"What it boils down to," Denton said, flipping the wipers off, "is they have scratched you from the list of competitors at the Southeastern Relays."

"What?"

"That's it. Now, please don't ask me to make any sense out of it. I am simply reporting the facts. Apparently there is no rationale behind it except, uh, you know, getting back at you."

"Are you serious about this?"

"Very."

"They are not going to let me run?"

"Nope."

"Did they say why, *for Jesus goddamn Christ's sake?*"

"Now don't go taking it out on me. I'm just telling you what

Cornwall told me. For what it's worth, he doesn't like it any more than you. He didn't even know at first how they found out you were running in the thing. Then he figured Hairlepp or one of the guys at the *Sun* went running to Doobey when they got the advance lists of competitors. You know how objective the old fourth estate is when it comes to sports. Anyway, Doobey himself apparently has authorized a policy that says Quenton Cassidy will not be permitted to compete on Southeastern University's benighted track come hell or high water."

"My Lord in heaven." Cassidy sat looking miserably out the window at the wet fields. "Can they *do* this?"

"Who knows? They're doing it. I asked my lawyer friend, Jerry Schackow, what he thought about it, but he said he couldn't tell without doing some research. He said it presents an interesting question."

"Swell."

"Meanwhile, not to worry. Training goes full bore. I'm going to start coming out in the afternoons more often to keep tabs on your interval work. You concentrate on the running and let me worry about getting you onto the track."

But Cassidy was despondent. He sat with arms folded, shaking his head in disbelief as he watched the fields and scrub forests pass. They finally reached Art's Steakhouse at the edge of town. Denton slapped him on the knee jovially.

"All right now, let's get us some dinner and try to think pleasant thoughts. I might even have an Irish whiskey myself."

"I wouldn't recommend it," Cassidy said glumly. "It seems to conjure up evil humors."

BRUCE DENTON rarely disclosed all he knew at one time. With Cassidy he preferred to let important information come in dribbles, as if by accident. He knew intuitively that such intelligence, invested with self-discovery, retained hard lines in a sometimes blurry world.

But as to his courageous attempt to intervene with higher authority—no less than Old Man Prigman himself—he chose to say nothing at all. Not that he was embarrassed by the comic futility of his effort; but he now realized the true nature of his adversary and decided to keep his own counsel while considering new tactics. He schemed with the controlled joy and abandon of a supposedly reformed street fighter suddenly finding himself in a brawl not of his own making.

He had gained his audience with Prigman in a very practical manner: he made himself an extremely good-natured pest. He sat around the waiting room reading old copies of *Florida Rancher,* grinning cheerfully at Roberta, cracking his gum like a blissful field hand. The secretary, who liked her office uncluttered, could not handle it; when she typed three errors in the same sentence in an obsequious letter to the governor, she calmly got up from her desk, marched into the inner sanctum, and pleasantly demanded action. Once in the door, Denton (had he not known better) might have thought Steven C. Prigman had been sitting around for hours in delightfully sweaty anticipation of his arrival.

"Bruce Denton!" Prigman wrung his hand heartily. "Now this is a surprise!"

"How do you do, sir?" Denton smiled despite himself. Why can't they deal with this man? he thought.

"I hope you received my telegram after your wonderful victory."

"Oh yes, sir, it was one of the first to arrive," Denton lied happily. This was going to be easier than he thought.

"Fine, fine. You know, I've been meaning to have you and Jennifer over for dinner one night, but . . . this job!" He tossed his hands, a man who could only hope those folks he truly liked could understand why he had such scant time for them. Denton wondered who the hell Jennifer was.

"Of course, sir, I know how terribly busy you must be, so I wouldn't presume upon your time unless . . ."

"No problem! No problem at all, my boy. I have all the time you need." To prove as much, he glanced nervously at his watch. "So, what is it I can do for you?"

"Well sir, it concerns a young man named Quenton Cassidy . . ."

Prigman's face drooped so noticeably that Denton stopped, surprised. So Prigman was in on it.

"Oh," said the old man quietly, settling back in his chair.

"Yes, sir. I understand that he is not being allowed to participate in the Southeastern Relays next month and—" Prigman squirmed in his chair, an adolescent movement, full of irritation and not at all in character.

"Might I inquire," he interrupted Denton, "as to the reason for your personal concern in this matter?" He had shifted, in the subtle manner of Southerners of his species, from diplomacy to advocacy, disguising the maneuver with such sincerity and deference as to leave the object of his charm, whether hostile witness or cautious subordinate, unsuspecting until it was too late.

"Well sir, Mr. Cassidy is a friend of mine. I have been helping him with his training for some time now, and I feel he might be an outstanding competitor, perhaps even of Olympic caliber, given the right opportunities. I can't understand what possible reason there might be—and I know about the recent, uh, difficulties—possible reason, that is, for keeping him out of the upcoming—"

"Now, Bruce—may I call you Bruce?—this whole affair has been extremely unfortunate for everyone concerned. Extremely unfortunate. But I'm sure that you, being an athlete yourself, must understand that insubordination must be dealt with firmly. Now, I know some mistakes have been made—on both sides—

but in the final analysis, rules are rules. Perhaps your sport is somewhat different, being individual and all, but on the playing field there must be a supreme commander, a leader who must make life-or-death decisions right on the spot. A game can be won or lost on a split second's hesitation. There is no other way to function, my boy. If you had to gather a football team together to take a vote on every play, why there would be chaos! Anarchy! Pretty soon the cheerleaders would want a vote too! This democracy stuff just won't cut it on the gridiron, my boy. Now in track and field, I don't know—"

"Sir, respectfully, I don't think anyone has suggested anything of the kind. If someone had taken the time to talk with Mr. Cassidy, they would have seen he was not advocating, nor anyone else who signed the petitions, anything other than stopping petty harassment and invasion of privacy of the athletes—"

"It's all a matter of discipline! Following orders! Dick Doobey may not have been right all the time, but he was still Dick Doobey! The general. He gave orders. And then what happened? *Petitions!*" He said it as if pronouncing the name of some loathsome disease that had just claimed a loved one.

"I suppose," said Denton very quietly, "that I just don't happen to subscribe to the militaristic sports metaphor. I don't believe that a football field or a basketball court are battlefields, except to the most simplistic and unenlightened observers. Even granting the analogy, I don't think a general at war would go out and order his army to eat shit just for the hell of it. Sir."

Denton had a vague notion he was no longer being listened to. *Sports and religion in the Deep South,* he thought. When his last remark got no discernible response, he knew his time was up. Prigman was concerning himself with the lighting of a huge cigar.

"Well," the old man said at last, turning slightly to the side so as to look out his window across the windswept plaza. "At any rate, such insubordination and dissension cannot be tolerated among athletes. You have no idea the damage this whole affair has caused, not just to team morale, but to this university. I'm speaking in terms of our image among the people of the state of Florida. No idea."

Denton stood before the giant desktop, looking across at the gray, dapper old politico behind it. He had thought that surely sweet reason could be brought to bear, that somewhere an appeal might be fairly heard. But then, Denton was unencumbered by the knowledge of Steven C. Prigman's illustrious career as a jurist, and therefore was not prepared to meet an intellect capable of operating almost wholly in a bygone century.

"Sir, Quenton Cassidy has represented this institution honorably and well. He has been the Southeastern Conference mile champion for two years and the captain of his team. He holds numerous school records. He has a chance to truly excel now, and keeping him out of this track meet can serve no reasonable purpose whatsoever except—"

"I take issue with that," said Prigman, exhaling aromatic blue smoke. "You say that the boy might become a real blue-chipper, eh?"

"Well, we don't use that term in running, but yes, he might very well become—"

"Well, he shall not do so using the facilities of this university." Very final-sounding, this last.

"I was going to say: 'except possibly for revenge of some kind,'" Denton said sadly.

"Mmmm." Prigman was shuffling papers on his desk, impatiently. Denton started for the door. "Your committee chairman, Dr. Branum," Prigman said suddenly.

"Yes, sir?" Prigman was looking away from him, as if distracted by something out the window.

"Dr. Branum is very anxious for you to finish that dissertation quarter after next. You wouldn't want to get too involved in other matters and let that work slide, would you?" Denton considered simply walking out, but decided to stop. *All right, little man, have it your way. But I'm going to go to school on you now,* he thought. With a crooked smile he turned back to Prigman.

"No, sir! I guess I'd better keep my nose to the old salt mine."

"Fine, fine." Prigman was relighting his cigar, his mind obviously already on other treachery.

Denton thought, My Lord in heaven.

32.

The Interval Workout

AN INTERVAL WORKOUT," Cassidy once explained to a sports-writer, "is the modern distance runner's equivalent of the once popular Iron Maiden, a device as you know used by ancient Truth Seekers." Although overdistance laid the foundation, intervals made the runner racing mean. Quenton Cassidy liked them. Others preferred bamboo splinters under their nails. Cassidy figured that a natural affinity for interval work was the difference between those who liked to race and those who liked to train. And there is a difference. Racers express little enchantment with training for its own sake.

An interval workout is simply a series of fast runs of a specified distance in a specified time with a specified rest. The variables are limited only by the imagination of the coach and the physical limitations quickly apparent in his athletes (it is one thing to write "Ten quarters in 58 seconds with a 220 jog" and quite another to carry out those instructions). While a ten-mile overdistance run might be generally thought of as a pleasant diversion, very few of Cassidy's teammates thought of intervals as anything but a grueling ordeal, satisfying at best, horrifying at worst. It was precisely the kind of training, he knew, that tempered the body for racing. Though the distance runner is constantly striving for aerobic efficiency, the race itself is primarily an anaerobic experience. Everyone, the winner in his painful glory as well as the loser many seconds behind in his equally painful anonymity, suffers the physical bankruptcy of total oxygen debt. And since interval training is usually sharp enough to bring the runner to grips with oxygen debt very quickly in the workout, he learns to deal with the debilitating fatigue from the first repetition on. Other sports use an abbreviated form of interval training called "wind sprints," but where football and basketball players run 30 or 40 yards and take several minutes' rest between each, the miler will run 220 yards, 440 yards, a half mile or even three quarters of a mile at a time. Each second of his minute or two-minute rest period is sweeter than life itself.

It was little wonder Bruce Denton took more interest in Cassidy's interval training than in anything else that made up his 140 miles a week. At the beginning of March, Denton began to come to the cabin on interval days, sometimes spending the night; after running early with Cassidy in the morning, he would drive directly to his lab. If such a program had a deleterious effect on his marriage, he never mentioned it to Cassidy.

"I HOPE YOU LISTENED to me and took an easy day yesterday," Denton said as they jogged to the field.

"Okay, consider me psyched out. What's the program?"

"Twenty quarters in sets of 5, 110 jog between the quarters,

440 jog between the sets, 62- to 63-second effort but no watch as usual. That's it. For now."

Cassidy was surprised. It was a tough workout, but nothing he had not done many times before. Denton had been talking ominously about this one for days, and now the runner actually felt a little let down. With Denton he never knew what to expect. When weeks earlier he had instructed Cassidy to let his hair grow and not to shave, Cassidy made it a point not to act surprised. He had his suspicions, but he also knew that Denton was not about to tell him any more. If he had wanted Cassidy to know, he would have told him already. Now the sun-bleached curls were around his ears and his chin had sprouted, of all things, a reddish beard which Cassidy was now becoming rather fond of. He pictured himself a gaunt Viking.

When they got to the field, Cassidy removed his shoes and joined Denton in some striders to loosen up. It was a gloriously clear, warm day and soon the shirtless runners were wringing wet with perspiration. Although he knew few runners who did so, Cassidy loved training barefooted. Denton considered it an aberration, but since it seemed to cause no complications, he tolerated the practice.

There had been, in fact, a few world-class runners who competed barefoot on the track and seemed no worse for it; and then there was Abebe Bikila who, incredibly, ran the twenty-six-plus miles of the marathon barefooted at the Rome Olympics, winning easily. There were arguments pro and con about whether it could be helpful in training or racing, but Cassidy just did it because he liked it. It allowed him to be closer to the grass, the soil, closer to the deepest hidden yearning of the runner: *to fly naked through the primal forest, to run through the jungle*.

They began. The first two or three always seemed somehow especially bad. Actually that was misleading. They seemed sluggish because the body was shocked by such a sudden demand for sustained speed. The heart rate shot up to the hummingbird levels it would have to maintain for some time. The legs became prematurely heavy, and the central nervous system sent up the message that such punishment could not be endured. But the central nervous system is overridden, of course, the runner knowing far better by now than his own synapses what his body can and cannot be expected to do. The runner deals nearly daily in such absolutes of physical limitations that the nonrunner confronts only in dire situations. Fleeing from an armed killer or deadly animal, a layman will soon find the frightening limits that even stark terror will not overcome. The runner knows such boundaries like he knows the sidewalks of his own neighborhood.

After the shock of the first several quarters, Cassidy settled into the pleasant, nearly comfortable rhythm of the workout, where each interval, though difficult, felt very much like the one before and the one to follow. After they finished the first set of five, the quarter-mile jog prescribed by Denton seemed almost too luxuriously long. During this time, once he had recovered his breath somewhat, Cassidy made a few remarks and generally tried to engage Denton in conversation; the older runner demurred, jogging on in what Cassidy thought a rather grim manner. They began the second set.

Round and round the field they went, each repetition so much like the one before they had to count out loud lest they forget how many they had done; Denton, the true compulsive, would assume they had done three rather than four and they would take a chance on doing an extra one. Cassidy, therefore, paid close attention to the tally. The only difference between one and the next was the slight increase in lactic acid in the lifting muscles on the top of the thigh that made each a little more difficult and started hurting earlier in the sprint. Otherwise, it was almost as easy to drift into the near-neutral mental state as it was on their long-distance runs. Denton was a perfect training partner; the pace did not vary more than half a second from one to the next.

In the third set Cassidy felt as though Denton was picking up
the pace, though it was unlikely. It simply required more effort
now to keep up the same speed. A miler, whose pace in a race
was quite a bit faster than sixty-three seconds, could still get a
lot out of such a workout. The key was not how fast he could run,
but how fast he could run while tired.

Cassidy did not allow himself to think of racing pace, for
these sixty-three-second quarter miles required so much effort it
would have been heartbreaking to think how much faster he
needed to run in an actual race. There were too many other fac-
tors: rest, a faster surface, and more important the incredible
psych he would build up prior to the race. Such comparisons
were not helpful and were dismissed quickly. In training it was
best to think about training. As he circled this little field twelve
miles from Kernsville on a Saturday afternoon, racing seemed an
exotic and glamorous activity indeed, the "trial" part of his Miles
of Trials.

Number fourteen was especially poignant. Finishing it, Cassidy rasped: "Eeeow, that one hurt!"

"Little. Fast." Denton gasped the words. Occasionally during
a repetition one of them would let his mind wander to a race,
long since run, and as the old memories seeped in, the pace
would inch up as adrenaline began surging involuntarily through
the system. The other runner would respond and soon they
would be flying around the worn path, racing different phantoms
from the past. The price for such a lapse was steep. They would
begin the next repetition still out of breath.

As bad as he felt at the end of the third set, by the time they
finished jogging their quarter, he was recovered. Denton's training usually called for very short recovery periods and Cassidy had
been amazed how he responded to the tiny snippets of rest. Recovery was the key; the faster one recovered, the faster he could
race. "A race," Denton would say, "is all go and no blow. So why
practice resting?"

The last set felt very much like the one before and when, at last, they finished number twenty, Cassidy let out a whoop. They had been running very hard for an hour. He looked over at Denton, expecting to see the happy relief that follows a hard workout, but Denton jogged on grimly.

"What now?" Cassidy asked cheerfully, thinking they would perhaps finish with some striders or a mile warm-down.

"Another twenty." Even though Denton said it seriously, Cassidy had to smile. After they did a few more strides and Denton did not dispel the grimness of his pronouncement, Cassidy knew he was serious. This, he thought, was a dirty trick.

And they began it all again. In their minds they took up each set separately, as if it were all they had to do. Five little quarter-mile circuits to be conquered, a mile and a quarter of hard running interspersed with those nearly cruel bits of rest, each quarter becoming in its own way a milestone, a feared and adamant obstacle that had to be dominated and put away so that its brother, now looming, could be faced. The sun was soon at tree level, splashing much of the field with dark cool shadows from the surrounding oaks. But for the desperate nature of their struggle, it would have been a remarkably pleasant scene; to the runners, however, it might just as well have been sleeting, so fierce was their attention to their toil.

Although as they finished the second set his legs were merely numb, Cassidy's arms and shoulders ached. When on occasion he slipped out of the trance to look at Denton, he saw no sign of unusual fatigue at all. This is how he puts the fear of God into them, he thought, he just keeps going and going like this.

They had both long since stopped speaking except to call out the number of the repetition as they finished, both of them gasping finally: "Twenty!"

The trees were now steeping in the beautiful dusty pink orange glow of sundown, the color of ripe mangoes filling the sky behind dark oaks. They jogged on, saying nothing; their deep hearty gasps echoed across the field. It did not really dawn on Cassidy until they were halfway around the field. By this time their breathing was getting back to normal, but they were still in considerable distress.

"Bruce, you're not going to . . . I mean, this is . . ." His voice faltered, weak with self-pity and resignation.

"Twenty more, Cass."

They jogged on quietly. Cassidy felt close to tears, and wasn't even ashamed about it.

"Bruce. Sixty quarters. Bruce, you can't be serious. Nobody does that kind of stuff anymore. Arthur Lydiard—"

"Screw Arthur Lydiard. Quenton, this is where you find out. This is the time and place. All the rest is window dressing."

"I don't know if I can do it."

"Quenton." He smiled for the first time all day. "You can do very nearly anything. Haven't you figured that out?"

"Yeah."

"Look, runners deal in discomfort. After you get past a certain point, that's all there really is. There is no finesse here. I know you can do this thing because I once did it myself and when it was over I knew some very important things."

"That you're a lunatic?"

"Maybe. Maybe we all are. But I expect you'll find out in your own way. That's why I'm going to let you do them by yourself, just the way people do everything that's important. You can slough off if you want, but by God, you'll sure as hell know when you're doing it, won't you?"

"I suppose," he said glumly.

"I'm going back to the cabin. I'll be back about the time you're finishing up."

"Swell."

C

HE BEGAN THE MELANCHOLY RITUAL as night was falling. After the first five he was running by the soft glow of a huge clear moon. Cassidy thought, Bruce thinks of everything.

Then he sought out the mental neutrality that is the refuge, the contained wan comfort of the runner. He grooved his mind upon the thin platinum rail of his task, a line that stretched out in front of him and disappeared into the gloom, further than he could contemplate all at once, even if he had the desire to, which he did not. When his trance broke and a word or phrase popped into his mind, his dizzy mind played with it like a seal with a beach ball, in a disturbing, gibberishly mad way, the way your mind acts in the druggy twilight before sleep. In a very controlled, abstract way, he knew how much he was suffering; the slightest break in his concentration allowed self-pity to well up in him instantly.

He was, in a manner of speaking, accustomed to this distress in the same manner that a boxer is "accustomed" to being struck; but the familiarity of experience in no way lessens the blow or mitigates its physiological effects. It merely provides the competitor a backdrop against which his current travail may be played, gives him a certain serenity and coolness in the face of otherwise overwhelming stimuli, allows dispassionate insight where otherwise there would be only a rush of panic. In a hail of killing blows, the fighter's quiet center of logic, schooled in brutality, will be calmly theorizing: We are hurt pretty badly. If we do not cover up and take up the slack we will soon be unconscious.

Not that this quiet center of logic particularly fears unconsciousness (indeed, how welcome it might seem at times), but it knows that one does not win while unconscious. In the same way, no highly trained runner slacks off because he fears the pain, but because the quiet center of logic tells him he will win nothing if he runs himself to a standstill.

All of this availed Quenton Cassidy not at all. His deeply

ingrained conditioning and his mahogany-hard legs merely allowed him to push himself that much more. He had the mental ability to literally run himself right into the ground like Sambo's tiger. He knew that Bruce Denton expected him to do exactly that, and, just as each repetition made the next seem more and more impossible, he knew that without question he *would* do it. There was no refuge in injury, his body could not be injured in this way. There was no refuge in mercy, there was nothing to forgive and no one to issue dispensation. And at last he saw: there was no refuge in cowardice, because he was not afraid. There was no alternative, it just had to be *done*.

He finished number seven, somehow running it too hard, which caused him to take deep and painful gasps and to spend a few seconds bent over grasping his knees before beginning his weak jog on to number eight (in his mind number three, and after that only two to go—beyond that he did not think). It was becoming harder and harder to get his breathing anywhere near normal in the 110-yard rest jog; he was starting the next interval gasping as if he had not stopped at all. Into the next one he charged, down the straight, around the turn, by a pine tree slashed in half by lightning (that to him meant only the halfway point), into the last turn, and then the last fifty yards of straightaway, legs, arms, shoulders, jawbone, ears, chest, fingers, all battling the strained numb pain of the lactic acid, all striving for that normality of motion that would preserve—should heaven and hell fall into each other in a cosmic swirl—the integrity of the stride. Let others flail; the runner runs truly to the end.

He finished and rasped, "Eight. You. Bastard."

But the ninth took special revenge, reduced him to such a level that he had to spend several seconds holding his knees and sucking in sweet but maddeningly unsatisfying air. When he finally trotted on, he looked up at the bright clear stars and his eyes welled, mixed with the hot sweat of his face, tears ran down to the spittle around his mouth and chin, and he felt quite literally that he was melting, turning to human slush as he jogged along. Only when he started a repetition did he become solid once more.

His mind had now taken up a melody, *Für Elise*, and played it constantly without apparent pattern except that as each new quarter mile began, so did his fragment of Beethoven; whereas the stars were cold specks of illuminated space dust to him, those haunting notes reassured that there were at least others in the universe capable of understanding. Each new quarter now began in a kind of physical sorrow and ended in nothing less than spiritual despair. He remembered suddenly the one marathon he had run. On the twenty-third mile he had looked around and discovered that everything seemed unfamiliar.

Convinced he was lost, he ran on like a forlorn child, blubbering and wailing. When he finished the race in 2:33 he saw he had been on the right course after all. But he still couldn't keep from weeping; he just didn't know why any longer.

After his fifteenth quarter he would have had to think for a moment to recall his own name. But now he had his full quarter mile of rest, that he took in mincing little steps, savoring every instant. His mind came out of neutral, reveled in giddiness. He was incredibly thirsty; his tongue was stuck to the roof of his mouth and he no longer had to spit out the thick white fluffs of congealed saliva; there was none. He dared not think of water, or of the first beer. Parched to the marrow, wobbly, near mad, he took his tiny jogging steps and waxed (so he thought) poetic:

> *Somewhere they fox-trot madly*
> *While in lunar shadows sadly*
> *I keep pace with crickets gladly*
> *And Moon rises with my bile*

Lord Godamighty, he told himself, launching into number sixteen (in his mind number one). *Für Elise* cranked up again and he wished it would go away. He hardly felt anything at all now. He hardly cared. As he was putting seventeen away, *Für Elise* degenerated into a kind of steam calliope gone haywire. Misplaced notes made what had been haunting, ugly; what had been precise and logical, mad and horrifying. As if to keep pace with the crumbling music, his form occasionally broke and an elbow would flap out wildly, a knee would catch its brother instead of sliding by. Poor Elise, he thought. Poor everyone.

Eighteen was a shambles. Nineteen required all his effort to keep the pace from slipping down to a stumble. It had fallen off badly during the last few sets, but there was nothing to be done about it. When he finished the nineteenth, he let out a slight, wild, but oddly unjoyous, whoop. He was vaguely aware that Denton had returned, but it quickly slipped his mind. His mind was devoid of any thought save finishing the last one.

On the last he simply sprinted away the life in him. The thin sliver of monorail that had once stretched out to forever now dropped off into a sheer abyss just over the horizon. Once more down the straight, around the far turn, past the pathetic half-pine, into the last turn, flailing now a little, and (all slow motion now), feeling each step of the last fifty yards until it was over.

He staggered about, tightly grabbing his knees, eyes clenched shut, painfully, for the tears could not get out, while the sweat seemed to seep in easily. Denton stood beside and held him steady, with a gentleness of a medic treating the newly wounded. And like a casualty, Cassidy seemed not to notice him.

Denton walked him back slowly, talking to him quietly all the way. Cassidy, still deep in his anguish, said nothing. Denton fed him from the blender, let him drink all the liquids he wanted, then gently put him to bed.

"Quenton, you—"

"I know," Cassidy said. His eyes were still moist; he turned away. "But it is a very hard thing to have to know."

Denton nodded, smiled at him as he swatted him once on the fanny (the muscles there were quivering, he thought, *just like it was for me*), and left. Cassidy was in a deep sleep by the time Denton was out the door.

Cassidy awoke only once during the night, filled the toilet with bloody urine (something Denton told him might happen), and went back to bed. He slept seventeen hours altogether and when he awoke at last, the runner, paragon of fitness and efficient mobility, *this* runner at least, had trouble getting around. He went back to bed.

33.

Orchids

I MUST HAVE HUMAN CONTACT," he told Denton. "And I'm not talking about your standard Newberry barmaid who mixes better metaphors than drinks."

"Chasing it," Denton said, "is more of a pastime than a runner can handle, generally speaking."

"Well, if you don't get me out of here among people who talk with recognizable syntax, I'm liable to do something rash, like set fire to your little dream retreat and then I hop a freight train."

And that is how Cassidy found himself at, of all things, a cocktail party, beginning to admit to himself a certain degree of social ineptitude of the variety that can culminate with your pants cuff inexplicably in someone's lemon meringue pie. Yet there it was: people clearly made him nervous.

Denton had abandoned him early in the evening—intentionally, he now suspected—and he had struggled through several conversations with guests who, though sincere and intelligent enough, gave off a carefully cultivated aura of university-town bohemianism. Though they would surely rise in the morning, gargle, and proceed to their offices to fill teeth, draw wills, grade papers, and otherwise keep the cogs of the republic whirring away, still they might at any moment (given the appropriate pep talk) grab a thirty-aught-six and a slab of jerky and take to the hills to fight the good fight. Most of it struck him as bizarre, and at the same time he was observing it, he was worrying about the fact that even after several days of light workouts, he still had not recovered fully from Denton's interval ordeal.

And he tired quickly of the standard party fare that goes: "You run twenty *miles?* Without *stopping?* I couldn't run twenty *feet,* har har har har . . ." He would have to bite his tongue to keep from saying that it had been real humorous the first thousand times he had heard it. He had forgotten what it was like, this thing with the stupid jokes. And too there were the questions: What did he eat? Did he believe in isometrics? Isotonics? Ice and heat? How about aerobics, est, ESP, STP? What did he have to say about yoga, yogurt, Yogi Berra? What was his pulse rate, his blood pressure, his time for the hundred-yard dash? What was the secret, they wanted to know; in a thousand different ways they wanted to know *The Secret.* And not one of them was prepared, truly prepared, to believe that it had not so much to do with chemicals and zippy mental tricks as with that most unprofound and sometimes heartrending process of removing, molecule by molecule, the very tough rubber that comprised the bottoms of his training shoes. The Trial of Miles; Miles of Trials. How could they be expected to understand that?

When he finally heard the one about how "I couldn't *drive* as far as you *run* . . ." he thought, *Death on a plate.* Fleeing to the kitchen, he was fishing around in the ice tub for a nondiet beer when he noticed that the dark-haired girl had followed him in.

She stood with one fist on her hip, watching him with faint amusement, but in a nice way, her head cocked curiously, and this: a flash of white carnivorous teeth against her dark face. I'm not up to this, he told himself.

He was fumbling around in the tub a little more than was called for and since he figured she was waiting for him to get his ass out of the way, he dived in with both hands and finally speared a normal beer. His hands were stiff and numb from the ice.

"Good old fattening kind," he said lamely *(oh aren't we just the conversationalist?).* He heh-hehed good-naturedly, wondering when he had become a total moron, and was about to make his hasty escape when she laughed. It was a remarkably unaffected laugh, throaty and real. It stopped him.

"You were not having much fun out there," she said. It was a statement, not a question. Then he noticed she already had a drink in her hand.

"I suppose not. Shows, huh?" He cracked the beer, dropped the tab into the ice, took a manly slug, and stuck his left hand into his back pocket to get it warm. He rocked back on his heels, looking about the kitchen as if truly absorbed by its contents. Maybe she's never seen anyone talk to the cookware, he thought.

"Would you like to see the orchids in the backyard?" she asked.

"Orchids? There are orchids in the backyard?"

"No." She laughed. "Not a one. Come on." She took him by the hand and led him back through the living room and out the sliding glass doors. There were no orchids. They sat on the far side of the pool on a child's swing set and listened to the noise of a party that now seemed somehow distant, faintly ludicrous. Cassidy wondered at first why it seemed so nostalgic, but then remembered, *There were grown-up parties long ago, and I sat in swing sets and listened to them.*

She was a psychology instructor, working on her Ph.D., and

she did not in the least want to talk about it. He judged her to be twenty-four or twenty-five, not as pretty as Andrea, but with her irony-ridden eyes and the amusement obvious in her forehead and eyebrows she might at any moment—he figured—have him sitting back on his haunches more or less barking like a seal. *Maybe I'm too easy,* he thought.

She was clearly a woman who could take care of herself and for some reason that rattled him.

"You must not go to parties much. At least I've never seen you around before," she said. Cassidy was drawing designs in the frost on his beer can.

"No, I suppose not. When you get right down to it, I don't really do much of anything."

"Except your running."

"Yes, except that."

"Doesn't sound very interesting."

"Oh hey"—he sat up straight—"it's not. Take my word for it." Deftly he watched her reaction and then in almost perfect sync repeated her next question right along with her:

"Then why do you do it?"

She remained unflustered however, laughed, and waited politely for his response.

"I wish there were some very clever, eminently acceptable answer to that. It's like when people ask me what I think about when I'm running. I usually say something like 'quantum mechanics.' Sometimes I say 'music.'"

"Music?"

"It's as good as any. Sometimes I *do* think about music. Actually when you're training you can think about anything you want, almost. But in a race, everyone thinks about the same thing."

"Which is?"

"The race, oddly enough."

"And what do you tell people who keep insisting on knowing why you do it?"

"I say it keeps me regular. Or I say I'm going out for the Olympics; they can sort of understand that since it's on the TV."

"You say it as if it were a joke."

"Oh, it's no joke, it's just that it's such a hard thing, such a slim chance; you have got to be so *lucky* even after you are so *good*. The odds are just against you, that's all. It's like a little kid landing the part of the carrot in his school play on nutrition, and having it go so well that his mother goes around telling everyone someday he'll win an Oscar. I mean, he might very well do it, but—"

"Bruce Denton did it," she offered.

"Bruce Denton won an Oscar?"

She gave him one of those one-knuckle female jobs to the deltoid that brought real tears to his eyes.

"Bruce Denton doesn't seem abnormal to you," he grunted, rubbing the spot painfully, "because he's walking around this very house munching pretzels and telling off-color jokes. But he's probably the only Olympic distance runner for a thousand miles. It is not a . . . normal thing to have one at your party, you know? It is not normal to . . . ah, never mind. It lacks perspective. And that hurt, by the way."

"Hmmm. So you spend all your time doing something admittedly boring that you have no good explanation for, and then when you go out to have a good time, you sit around looking like someone just shot your dog. Interesting."

"Think I'm a head case?"

"No doubt about it. Welcome to the Laughing Academy." She motioned in the general direction of the party, and as if on cue there was a wild burst of laughter and suddenly a man with his shirttails out went crawling on all fours by the sliding glass door at a startling clip. He was looking back over his shoulder and kind of slinking along. Cassidy recognized him as an ophthalmologist named Caldwell something who had earlier told him to "hang right on in there."

"Dr. Hodge," she said. "Coyote imitation. It's not too bad, actually. This is what's known as middle-class stoned."

Cassidy turned back, looked at her for several seconds, and really couldn't think of a thing to say. It occurred to him that he was a pretty dull guy. She reached over and touched his beard. The intimacy of the gesture was incredibly soothing to him.

"I like the new look. Very Nordic. Much different from those awful crew-cut pictures in the *Sun*. They must have been taken when you were a freshman. When did this come about?"

"Last few weeks. Bruce's harebrained scheme to get me into the relays in two weeks. That was one of the reasons he didn't want me to come tonight. Supposedly everyone here is sworn to secrecy. Actually, I think it's all a crock."

"Someone said something about it but I didn't pay much attention."

"I have been banned from competing on Southeastern University's benighted track, now and forevermore." He held up his hands, a preacher pronouncing benediction; then he burped politely behind his hand. Four beers was about his limit now. But he was beginning to feel pretty good about the evening after all. "Dangerous rabble-rouser that I am," he added. "Rabble, rabble, rabble."

"Let me ask you something," she said softly.

"Sure"—he finished the can with a flourish—"anything. Anything at all." She put her hand on his knee and ran a fingernail along the ridges on the outside of his thigh. It felt to her like nothing so much as a bunch of tightly bound bridge support cables.

"Did you think I was being brash in there, about the orchids and all?" Softly still.

"Uh."

"Well, did you?"

His Adam's apple felt like a soggy tennis ball.

"Does it surprise you?" She leaned over to capture his downcast eyes, led him back up to look at her. "Well?"

He hated his idiotic awkwardness, his painful lack of any kind of grace. He was a cloistered monk turned loose among Manhattanites, flap-flapping around in his scrungy sandals high up in the carpeted sky, nervously sipping some strange heady cocktail, preoccupied with his own alarming armpits and responding to the simplest inquiry like this: buh dee buh dee buh dee.

"You have to try to understand," he said miserably, still watching her dark serpentine hand, "I have no moves left. You have to try to understand how it is . . ."

"Oh." She smiled that carnivorous smile. "I will."

34

Pause . . .

F OR ME? You shouldn't have!" Cassidy said when Denton handed over the cardboard box. It was getting close and Denton had announced it was time for brass tacks.

"You don't know how unfunny that may be. No telling what kind of fiery crap will fill the air," Denton said. But his smile indicated his real degree of concern. As Cassidy opened the box Denton thought, *He really doesn't know what he's done; his lightest day was eight miles when he sprained his ankle that time.*

"Finnish national team sweats! They're beautiful." Cassidy held up the robin's-egg-blue top. The blue and white flag of Finland was in miniature over the left breast.

"I'd like them back in good condition please, Seppo, as I had to trade them straight up for a pair of USAs."

"Zeppo? Zeppo?"

"Seppo, ninny. Here is your contestant's entrance pass and your number. You are listed as Seppo Kaitainen, a miler from Finland currently competing for Central Ohio Tech. Nobody knows about it but you and me and the guy I got to send in the application and fee from Ohio. Cornwall snapped you right up, Seppo! It appears you have run yourself some outstanding times this year."

"I might have known it would be good and kinky."

"Kinky, hell! It's pure genius is what it is. You have no idea how much different you look from the old close-cropped anarchist of yore. You get yourself some wire-rims, garble up your English a little more than usual, ask for some pickled herring, and by God the sunbitches will think you're Paavo Nurmi."

Cassidy was holding the sweat top up to himself and trying to see himself in the window reflection.

"You honest to God think it'll work?"

"Fish tread water? Frog waterproof? Wild dog bay at the—"

"All right, all right. I sense a little pride of authorship here. What happens if someone catches on? Won't your man at Central Ohio Whatchamacallit get screwed over?"

"That illustrious center of higher learning doesn't exist, to my knowledge. Even if it did, there would be no one there to whom, as my counselor friend says, liability would attach. My buddy was only passing through when he mailed in the application. He is a proud resident of Illinois."

"All this to get into a goddamn track meet."

"Not just any track meet, Seppo old buddy, not by a long shot. It's not every day a Finn attending an Ohio school gets to run the world record holder from New Zealand right here in north Florida. You ought to can the skepticism and thank your lucky stars I was able to bring the whole production off."

Cassidy smiled. "Hey. I appreciate it, I really do. But since I have apparently made the traveling squad, I'm going to expect Central Ohio to spring for my varsity letter."

"Say no more, Seppo, we treat our foreign athletes right," he said as he stood. "Right now I've got to go see if I can salvage what's left of my marriage. I'll be out early and we'll talk strategy."

"Mmmm." Cassidy's mind was off someplace and Denton hoped it was not out on the track, thrashing himself through it again.

"Hey . . . Hey! Leave it alone for a while. Get some sleep; you might want to take some of that mild nerve stuff in the cabinet. Try to keep your mind off it as much as possible. You know all about this stuff." He started for the door. "Oh, there's a nondescript racing vest in the box in case you don't have one. Seppo wouldn't be racing in his national colors, it's just a plain—"

"Bruce, is there any . . . I mean, could there be any conceivable way I might could win this thing? Seriously, I mean?"

Denton stopped. "Hells bells, Quenton. You can put the fear of God into him, I know that. But give yourself some time. You don't have to go out and trounce the best guy in the world just because you've done some great training here. Let him pull you along to a super time." He started for the door again but stopped with his hand on the knob.

"You know those demons of yours you're always talking about? Well, Walton's got armies of them. You can see them in his eyes when he warms up, scrambling around just wailing and carrying on."

"Well," Cassidy said, standing and stretching, "I guess we just let the fiery little bastards loose and at each other."

Denton opened the door, looked back before leaving.

"Was there ever any other way?"

THE NEXT NIGHT after dinner they sat on the front porch right as the sun was going down, sipping coffee and staring into the darkening oaks; fireflies winked in the deeper woods and a red-tailed hawk circled once high overhead and silently floated away to some far-off haven, leaving the chilled deep blue of the sky to the earlier stars. There was an unmistakable feeling of something large having passed and something large coming: eye of the hurricane.

Cassidy held his mug with both hands and moved closer to the barbecue grill, where coals glowed pale orange, and thought, The adults would sit on the porch like this while we caught fireflies and played tag on the front lawn. The older of his North Carolina cousins would grow irritable and little Quentie would be counseled not to remain so long uncaught.

Only children and dogs, it seemed, were supposed to run, and they all shared the sidewalks. Perhaps that accounted for Cassidy's growing sense of unreality out in the cabin. He no longer could claim his activity was an adjunct to scholastic pursuits, a schoolboy's preoccupation. He was now beyond that, but where? A professional in a field where there was no profession? The horrendously physical nature of his days and ways occasionally caused him to stir; intellectual grist of late had been confined to mind candy of the *Lord of the Rings* variety. He had begun to wonder how much of this was really necessary.

You feel like an animal? Denton had asked. Just what Elliott told Cerutty when he wanted to quit. (As if that were some kind of answer.) But there was a day, Denton said, when Cerutty had been caught in a riptide at Portsea, and Elliott had grabbed the old man by his white hair and just swam. He swam and swam, not going anywhere at all, just there in place, for what seemed like hours, *until the fucking ocean just gave up.* Animal's exactly right, Denton had said, but *Jesus, what an animal.*

Then Denton had looked over at him and said: "Let's go run."

And Quenton Cassidy, having not a thing else in the world to do, said okay. So ended the great intellectual revolt of March.

It was shortly after that Cassidy began to notice something very strange in his training: it had become nearly impossible to make himself hurt. His ten miles in the morning left him only flushed and hungry; in the afternoon he thrashed himself through his distance run or interval workout and finished feeling itchy, like something was going on. So he told Denton about this strange sensation of invulnerability and admitted to being puzzled.

But the Olympian just settled back against the porch step, sipped on his coffee, and smiled warmly at the miler.

"How nice," he said, "for you to have arrived right on time."

Now within forty-eight hours, he would be lacing very tightly those thin kangaroo-skin slippers with pin spikes and he would attempt to overtake the most locomotively efficient Homo sapiens to yet tread the earth. At the distance of one mile, that is. Among all the swift messengers of the Hellenistic era, among the Masai warriors of the plains of Africa who laughingly run game to the ground, among the mustachioed old professional runners of the lunatic marathon-dance age who ran for large purses, among all these there was not one who even approached this modern, black-suited New Zealander; the first human to run faster—not than four minutes—but than three minutes and fifty seconds, a barrier without quite the symmetrical poetry for mankind perhaps, but one with such a terrible message for other runners—those who knew best how to interpret such messages— that they wobbled. Some gave up in despair, some sought refuge in other events. Liquori, it was said, went to 5000 meters.

Bruce Denton, sipping his coffee quietly, knew well the carnivorous nature of prerace fears. He sought to relieve what he felt was an ominous silence. The one thing he did not yet know about the miler was his control. Denton feared that during the next few hours the runner, like an aging automobile on a country road, might simply rattle himself to pieces.

"There was the Englishman Oates," he said, "on an expedition to one of the poles, I forget which. Out of supplies and fuel, the men were sitting around in a tent while a deadly blizzard raged. Several, I believe, had already frozen to death. Oates, deciding to end it all, rose and announced: 'I'm going outside. I may be some time.'"

Cassidy smiled over the top of his mug, the coffee now going lukewarm in the chill of the evening, and counted that as the moment he most loved Bruce Denton.

"It's all right, Bruce," he said. "Really. It's all right."

35

The Orb

S AYING SOMETHING about walking off his macaroni and cheese, Cassidy escaped to the evening. There was a bit of marital uneasiness in the air, a strain that he may have had more than a little to do with, but for now all he could think of was closing the glistening, seamless orb, receptacle of his fiercest yearning.

In the afternoon they had gone to a deserted high school track for the last session, a nearly light-headed tune-up; for the first time in months he was completely rested and strong and when Denton walked over and held up the watch grimly it said 24.8. That was the fourth and final 220. Denton shook his head disgustedly.

"I couldn't help it," Cassidy said.

"Okay," Denton replied; he would have liked to have been able to show a little genuine anger at such a reckless display, but he knew how it felt and so remained quiet as they jogged a final slow mile around the battered old asphalt track.

During dinner there was none of the usual banter and Jeannie, after trying several times to relieve the tension, finally clammed up, allowing everyone to stew in the awful clink-clank, chomp-chomp of nonconversing diners who, when the pressure is on, cannot seem to keep their silverware and their own mastication under control. It was nerve-racking for Denton and his wife, but Cassidy hardly noticed.

Now he was walking quickly, inexorably, toward the place he would complete the orb, set it gently adrift, and leave it hard and shining until it was time.

It was one of the early balmy spring evenings in Kernsville when no one wanted to go inside. The campus was bustling; the lighted tennis courts were full and other players sat around waiting patiently, talking and laughing. Groups of three or four made their way on foot to the student union or the nearer taverns, loaded cars roared to and fro, cyclists whirred by like mechanical butterflies, books and Italian sandwiches strapped onto luggage racks.

It was the kind of scene Cassidy would have reveled in before, but the roar was now a tiny faraway buzz in his skull, growing by the minute, and as he walked on consumed by it, he was aware only that scenery was moving by as always, steadily and without apparent effort. He walked with the light, brisk, slightly pigeon-toed gait of an athlete, and though he walked very quickly, his breath would not have troubled the smallest candle. He took in even, deep measures of cool air with mechanical regularity, disinterestedly feeling inside his chest the huge heart muscle thumping its slow liquid drumbeat. His legs coiled and uncoiled with rhythm; sacks of anacondas. That part of it was done as well as he could humanly do it. Now he would see to the rest. He had made this pilgrimage many times before and though he would probably do so many times again, he never quite got over the eerie feeling that each time could be the last. Soon he was on the far side of campus where there were few dormitories and hence less activity, fewer lights, and none of the happy spring weekend noise.

Moths fluttered around the single streetlight as he went through the gate, and though the rubdown smell of wintergreen and sweat was as familiar to him as the musky woodiness of his old room at Doobey Hall, his heart still jumped. The usual night joggers were out, and if they cast haughty glances at this mere stroller on their turf, the stroller paid no attention. He walked clockwise around the curve to the starting post at the beginning of the first turn, and stood there a few feet behind the parabolic bend of the starting stripe. He looked around and tried to imagine, in Hollywood-style flashes, the skeletal bleachers full, the now dark klieg lights burning down, the pageantry of the multi-hued sweat suits from a thousand schools flashing by as athletes warmed up. He would be part of that faceless panorama too, until the announcement over the loudspeaker that never failed to twist his heart around with a spurt of adrenalized fear: "FIRST CALL FOR THE MILE RUN." The all-consuming roar, the overwhelming psych would begin then and would build up until he stood ready on this line, at once controlled and near lunacy, fearless and terrified, wishing for the relief of the start, the misery of the end. Anything! Just let the waiting be done with! Cassidy toed the starting line there in street clothes and was able to get some of it: a few of the runners would jog back and forth in their lanes, some would jiggle their fingers, some would jump up and down (all this more habitual than thera-peutic). The orange-sleeved starter would walk among them with his pistol, saying, *"All right, gentlemen, all right."* He would talk gently, trying to somehow ease things for them, hoping to pre-vent a false start by calming them with the soft modulation of his voice. They were not as bad as sprinters, he knew, but they were still pretty skittish. The runners would gather nervously at the starting line, taking care not to look one another in the eye.

The starter would say: "There will be two commands, gentle-men, 'take your marks' and then the gun. All right, gentlemen, stand tall. Stand tall, gentlemen." He would sound a little like an executioner.

And Cassidy stood tall there in the dark, while a cool breeze ruffled the ragged lock of hair on his forehead, knowing that for that one instant there would be a kind of calm in the midst of all that pounding, roaring furor, a moment of serene calm before an unholy storm. There would be a single instant of near disbelief that it would finally be happening in a fraction of a second; finally happening after the months, the miles, the misty morn-ings; finally happening after the eighth or ninth now forgotten interval along the way somewhere that broke your heart once again. He would be leaning over tensely with the rest of them while the white lights burned down on them and for an awful split second he would feel as if his legs had no strength at all. But then his heart would nearly explode when the pistol cracked. Cassidy felt a little of that now. He took a deep breath and began walking into the first turn, counterclockwise, the way of all races.

The first lap would be lost in a flash of adrenaline and pound-ing hooves. They would crash into the first turn in a bunch; the technical rule was that with a one-stride lead, a runner could cut in front. As with many such rules it was honored generally in the breach; the real-life rule of the first turn is exactly this: every man for himself. He would run powerfully into this turn, Cassidy thought, just like always, and he would use his elbows if he needed to make some space. Cassidy walked the turn, trying to imagine the sudden rasping of heavy breathing, the flashing of elbows and spiked feet all around. You had to be calm in the heavy traffic, he knew, hold back your impatience and control the panic; wait for opportunities. The first lap would be like that the whole way: fast, scary, with no pain or serious effort. The rampaging adrenaline and pent-up energy did that. The first lap was a process of burning it off; no one ever won a mile race on the first lap. Cassidy walked the far, dark straightaway. On the opposite side from the main bleachers, it was the loneliest part of the track. This was where the race-acute senses picked up the single calls of encouragement (usually from teammates), sometimes the idiotic suggestion called out by those who knew no better ("pick it up, pick it up"). There would be the occasional giggling of moronic teenyboppers who did not quite know what they were laughing about. But those were the peripheral toys of a frenzied mind; the real work of the shining orb was monitoring the steadily droning *pocketa-pocketa* of a human body hurtling along at a constant fifteen-plus miles an hour. He walked through the far turn and up the straight to the starting post. Someone would be reading out times, probably around fifty-seven or fifty-eight, assuming that no one went crazy during the first quarter. You'll hear the crowd again along here, he thought, particularly after we go through under sixty; they won't be cheering for some goddamn Finn, but you'll hear them just the same.

Whether a psychological thing or not, the second lap was when it always hit him, either right at the post or as they rounded the turn. The shocking enormity of the physical effort descended on him then and he knew from there on in it would be pretty grim business. At this point the carefully nurtured mental toughness, tempered by hours of interval work, would allow him to endure the shock to his system and race on. He would be ready for it and he would know it was going to get far worse. He could be the best-conditioned athlete in the world, but if his mind was not ready to accept the numbing wave at the start of the second lap, he would not even finish, much less hope to win.

Cassidy walked through the turn, and again into the lonely back straight. By this time he would be concentrating on pace, not allowing himself to become frightened by the first hint of numbness and discomfort. It wouldn't be "pain" exactly, not at this point, but it would not be altogether pleasant either. It was here the pace might tend to slow, something he would have to watch, something he would damned well prevent if he had to. He would now go into his floating stride, the long ground-eaters, and he would think to himself: cover territory.

No one ever won a race on the second lap either but plenty of people lost them there. This would be the time for covering distance with as little effort as possible. Through the far turn and into the home straight again he tried for the feeling and thought he got it pretty well. Finally around at the starting post again he tried to get the awfulness of the start of the third lap, but could not. He had seen the drawn haunted look on his own face in mid-race photographs and still he could not get that feeling; it was contained there somewhere in the glistening orb, he knew, and would never get out. Denton was right about it, you could think about it all you want but you couldn't feel it until you were there again. He knew only that here, at the halfway point, he would be once again in extremis. It would flabbergast him to think (so he would do so only for an instant) that he was only halfway through it. He would have run the first half mile faster than he could run a half mile flat out in high school (1:59.2) and he would have a long way to go.

He walked into the turn of the third lap. Here the real melancholy began, when the runner might ask himself just what in the hell he was doing to himself. It was a time for the most intense concentration, the iciest resolve. It was here the leader might balk at the pain and allow the pace to lag, here that positions shifted; those whose conditioning was not competitive would settle to the back of the pack to hang on, the kickers would move up like vultures to their vantage points at the shoulders of the front runners. It was a long, cruel lap with no distinguishing feature save the fact that it had to be run. Every miler knows, in the way a sailor knows the middle of the ocean, that it is not the first lap but the third that is farthest from the finish line. Races *are* won or lost here, records broken or forfeited to history, careers made or ended. The third lap was a microcosm, not of life, but of the Bad Times, the times to be gotten through, the no-toys-at-Christmas, sittin'-at-the-bus-station-at-midnight blues times to look back on and try to laugh about or just forget. The third lap was to be endured and endured and endured.

Cassidy reached the home straight again, thinking, No matter how bad it is, I can't let it lag here, whatever the cost. If I have to lead the whole mothering thing, I can't let it lag here. Then he was walking back by the post for what would be the gun lap. As soon as the pistol cracked, he would feel a tingling on the back of his neck and the adrenaline would shoot through his system again. A quarter of a mile to go and he would become a competitive athlete again, looking around to size up the situation, leaning a little into his stride and once again, even through the numbing haze then gripping his body, feeling pride in his strength.

Cassidy walked through the turn, pumping his arms a little, thinking of the nervous crowd noises as the pace began to pick up. Perhaps there would be only a small group left in it now; three, four maybe. But they would all have ambitions; no one ever ran down the back straight of the gun lap with the leaders without thinking he had a shot at it. On Cassidy walked, along the lonely straight imagining the bristling speed as the pace heated up; there would be some last-second evaluations, some positioning and repositioning, and then finally the kicks, one by one or all at once, blasting away for the tightly drawn yarn across the finish line. Into the turn with only a 330 to go, *everyone* would be into it by then, everyone still in contention. Walton was known to kick from more than a 440 out, so surely his hand would be on the table. Coming out of the final turn just at the place Landy turned to look for the elusive Bannister, Cassidy walked into the final 110 straight and thought, Here, as they say, it will be all over but the shouting; you will fight the inclination to lean backward, fight to keep the integrity of the stride, not let overeager limbs flail around trying to get more speed, just run your best stride like you have trained ten thousand miles to do and don't for God's sake let up here until the post is behind you. The die would be cast here, and no praying or cheering or cajoling or whimpering would change it. He had lost in this final straight before, but not as much as he had won here; neither held much in the way of fear or surprise once you were there. Such matters, as Denton had often said, were settled much earlier: weeks, months, years before, they were settled on the training fields, on the ten-mile courses, on the morning workout missed here or made up there. Other than maintaining and leaning at the tape, Denton had told him, there is not much you can do about it. Heart has nothing to do with it. In the final straight, *everyone* has heart.

Cassidy walked on past the finish line, across which someone would hold the taut yarn and blink as the runners flashed by. It was still more than twenty-four hours away, but standing there in the calm anonymous night five yards past the familiar white post, Quenton Cassidy knew at that instant the depth of his frenzied yearning to feel the soft white strand weaken and separate against his heaving chest.

The demons were now in control; it no longer made him afraid.

36

The Race

THE NOISE from the stadium carried out here but Cassidy didn't pay much attention. He liked doing most of the warm-up ritual out on the cross-country course where he could think. The routine itself was automatic: four miles easy; then long, flowing striders, another mile easy, faster striders, then on with the spikes, some sprints on the track, then jog until time. It was the roar in his head he had to fight.

It had to be contained, suppressed, released only in that slow crescendo of calculated frenzy that would crest when the pistol cracked and he unleashed it all. The orb now floated gently in his mind, glistening, peaceful, hard as spun steel. It would hold all grief, all despair, all the race-woes of a body going to the edge; it would allow him to do what he had to do until there was nothing left.

Yes, he had decided long ago it was better to get ready out here, where things were quieter, more normal, more like his everyday routine. Trying to warm up in the stadium, being close to the crowd, would make him jittery, causing the roar in his head to build in spurts, getting him there too early. It might upset the orb and when the despair descended on him he would have no place to put it. Or he might be in such a lunatic state as to turn the first 220 in twenty-five seconds out of sheer scream-ing hysteria. No, it was better out here, where it was quiet, where he could get ready in the same way he had done all the rest; it gave some comfort, this last bit of tranquility.

He jogged slowly by the married-student housing area, watching little children play under the trees. It was the eerie, almost magic, postdinner hour when time stands still for a child, when all existence floats in a cool gray bath of dying day and Order is mercifully drawn from a chaotic infinity by a mother's come-home call.

"Erica! Jeremy!" Two little figures scuttled away in the shad-ows. He was getting farther and farther from the stadium, but he had plenty of time. Some other runners passed in pairs and threes, but no one spoke. One nodded at Cassidy but looked puz-zled. What would they be thinking about this bearded Finn with the ragged blond hair?

Would they think they recognized him from some *Track & Field News* photo?

Cassidy jogged on. It was early-May warm and subtropical flowers ruled the air dizzily: the kind of evening so heavy with promise as to make him wonder if his life could ever be quite the same again as it was now, while he was so vital, so quick, so nearly immortal; while his speed and strength were such that he could be called out by only a handful of men on earth. Surely there could not be that many of us walking around like this, he thought.

He felt a strange brand of nostalgia now that it was so close; a nostalgia for this moment, for this next hour. The present was so poignant he had begun to reminisce already. He thought of Michelangelo's *David* pondering the stone: David wondering too if life would ever be the same.

He was about to go to the edge, had every bit of the where-withal to *get* to the edge. The inevitability of his journey there was never very far from his mind now; he knew that before too very long he would be in mortal distress.

The time you won your town the race, we chaired you through the marketplace, he thought. Then a burst for twenty yards just to enjoy the sensation of sudden unleashed speed. He felt both flushed and tired. That was common. You never really know how you feel, he thought, until the second lap. Sometimes not even then. Sometimes you don't even know until the last lap, *the stiller town.*

When he reached Lake Alice, he slowed to a walk and then stopped altogether. He stretched out on the grass and did hurdles and butterflies. Stretching was always a pleasant indulgence.

Then he undid the vertical zippers along the legs of his warm-ups and felt up and down both Achilles tendons. All the knots and lumps were gone. Soft trails, he thought; goddamn Denton and those beautiful soft trails. He had made it through the winter okay, only two colds and no real injuries. He was a man without an alibi.

Two runners in Villanova sweats went by, but he didn't recognize either of them. From far off the crowd yelled as someone cleared a height or broke the tape in a sprint preliminary, and his own body responded by dumping a shot of adrenaline into his system. He caught it quickly. Not yet, he thought, not even close yet.

It was a time for daydreams; the roar in his head was far off now and building, but it would grow on its own. The problem now was control.

There had been a local race a long time ago, a five-miler late in the summer. As the runner tooled along the bicycle path on the Palm Beach side of Lake Worth he was sweating profusely; it flew off in arcs on every stride. True, he was not in very good shape yet, but it was far too early to worry about it. It was still summer and deathly hot.

The child stopped him right in his tracks. It was about a mile after he had made the turn at the Sailfish Club. The kid could have been no more than six or seven, and as he walked toward the runner, it was apparent there was something wrong with him; he moved without flow, all angles and juts. The runner thought: he's so pale. But the child was just beaming. Wispy hair fell back into place as the hot wind blew through it, clear blue eyes stared at Cassidy without fear or self-consciousness. Cassidy stood gasping, dripping puddles of sweat onto the asphalt. He tried his best to beam back. Through his gasping he couldn't help chuckling at how silly this was.

"Hello," Cassidy said.

"Hello," the child said happily. "What are you doing?"

"I'm running a race. What's your name?"

"Allan." The child laughed, put a small hand to his mouth, so thin as to seem transparent. The runner looked over his little legs for braces but saw none. The left shoe, however, seemed bulkier on the bottom than the other.

"A race?" The child laughed again, obviously wary of being teased. "But where are your opponents?" He said it "oh-po-nuts."

"Oh." The runner gestured back toward the Sailfish Club. "They'll be right along." The child cocked his head in a very curious, nearly feminine manner, but he was still beaming.

"You," he said, "run like a big cat." The runner swallowed.

"You," Cassidy said, "are the finest fellow I have run across all morning, Allan. And I guess I'd better be getting along before my oh-po-nuts come along."

"Good-bye, big cat."

"Good-bye, Allan."

As he slipped off and gathered speed, he looked behind every few yards to see the child still watching; finally he disappeared behind a curve of high hibiscus a quarter of a mile down toward the bridge. Wonder what he will think when the rest of them come clomping along, he thought. And although he really wasn't in very good shape yet he turned a 4:45 for the last mile, changed from his racing flats and jogged across the bridge toward home before the rest of them got in. If there was a medal or something they would just have to mail it to him.

For a long time after that he wondered what it was about that child.

A shriek from the stadium brought him back. He braked his wildly skittering heart.

CASSIDY SWOOPED INTO A STRIDER, held it until the speed built to racing pace, held it, held it, then eased off, slowed to a stride, then a jog, and finally to a walk a hundred yards away. He was on the flat grass in the field across the street from the stadium; other athletes flashed by in blurs of color. He allowed himself some excitement on one of the striders and instantly felt the goose bumps on the back of his neck. He hadn't ever had it quite this bad before.

The noise from the stadium across the street added to the growing roar in his head but it didn't matter now; it was all right now. He allowed it to come, let it fuel his stride as he started up, slipped into it, and then built up speed until his legs seemed to come detached from him and he flew along without conscious effort. Other athletes were at it too, nervous, casting furtive glances at one another (never looking anyone in the eye). A lot of people talk themselves right out of races now, Cassidy thought. He looked at his watch: 7:38. The mile was scheduled for 8:20 but they were running behind. Still, a few minutes later he heard the call over the loudspeaker: "FIRST CALL

FOR THE MILE RUN." His heart twisted around in his chest like a wild animal; it was an absolutely wrenching shot of adrenaline. *They were going to run it after all! He was going to have to go through with it!*

Then he got control again and steadied himself. Of course he was going to run this race. Take it easy. It was time to get into the infield and get used to being inside there, do the last touchups, put on the spikes: ritual, ritual, ritual. Then the last sprints, the final psyching. *Jesus,* he thought suddenly, *why am I doing this? I ought to be in the three-mile. I've been doing all that bulk work and everything. I can't possibly be ready for a mile* . . .

Then he steadied himself again; he thought of the last 220 the evening before and told himself: easy. He took a deep breath and walked over to pick up his bag. He had not spoken one word to anyone during the entire hour he had been out here. Runners flashed by. Everyone looked fast and fit as hell.

Then he caught himself again. Any of these mothers runs 3:58 in a goddamn time trial in the dead of night and he'll damned well deserve to eat my lunch. Again he told himself: *easy.*

Inside the stadium a 178-pound lad who could bench-press 300 pounds planted a 16-foot fiberglass pole in a tin box, inverted himself, and was tossed into the air a little more than 17 feet, 8 inches. When the crowd reacted to this feat with a roar, something flipped in Quenton Cassidy: his heart jumped so hard he thought his head was going to pop right off. The tumult in his head was like the roar at the bottom of a waterfall. He walked to the competitors' entrance and for a split second had a rush of ordinary civilian panic as well. He had forgotten completely about this disguise business.

But the little round face looked up from the clipboard and the cold stump of cigar went round and round.

"Well, let's see here, 242, why, I guess that would be you, Seppo! Go right on in there, boy, and you have yourseff a good race, yuh hear? Say, that ain't true what they say about you Finn boys drinkin' reindeer milk, is it? Didn't think so."

Cassidy heard Brady Grapehouse cackling behind him as he went into the stadium.

How the hell had Denton arranged that? he wondered. But then he was on the inside and the special atmosphere, the blue-white lights, the wintergreen-laced, multicolored carnival that is a major track meet sent his senses reeling, just as it always did. *God,* he thought. *Here I am again; here it all is and here I am with everything on the line one more time.* He looked back uptrack to make sure it was clear and then jogged across the lanes to put his bag down. His heart skittered again, feeling for the first time in weeks the springy Tartan beneath his feet. Officials were running here and there, hurdle setters scurrying around, timers checking watches. No one noticed the tall runner in robin's egg blue as he began the methodical jogging on the inside grass lane. The infield was a mass of motion. Javelin throwers were slogging back and forth in their strange sideways gait, hurling imaginary spears at their long-extinct enemies, broad jumpers bounded around, high jumpers took their run-ups, and the runners of all sizes circled the track in various stages of their warm-ups. It made a three-ring circus look like a quilting bee.

"SECOND CALL FOR THE MILE RUN." *Flash* went another shot of adrenaline through his veins—he took two gasping breaths that seemed wrenched from his body as if from one tossed suddenly into an icy sea. He got control again, this time with difficulty. Two laps, that's what the ritual called for. The roar inside his head drowned out the crowd altogether, except when they went wild over some performance. But Quenton Cassidy noticed nothing; he moved inside his own box. His gaze was starting to take on the trance quality, so that when he ran by Denton without seeing him, the older runner was not in the least surprised.

"Seppo!" he called. It took awhile to register. But then, of

course it was all right. Denton would know an international runner, it would only be natural. Denton held out his hand when
Cassidy circled back. He took it nervously.

"Sorry," Cassidy said. "He here yet?"

"Nope. But he will be. Best get your spikes on. How is it?"

"Banjo string. E-flat."

Denton nodded.

"Bruce, I can hardly swallow."

"It's okay. It'll be like all the rest once you get moving. Beforehand's tougher. I would jog with you but I don't want to push
our luck. Both Prigman and Doobey are here. Guess Walton's a
big enough attraction to draw even the football establishment.
Anyone say anything to you?"

"No. Guess it's working. I'll be all right. I want to do it alone
anyway." Denton noticed he was breathing fast, shallow, nearly
gasping. It was not important, he knew, so long as he had not
torn himself all up inside over it already. It would be all right
soon. He gripped Cassidy by the elbow.

"Cass, I . . ."

Cassidy looked Denton in the eye very briefly, then smiled.
He gripped Denton's forearm and held it hard for a moment.
Then he turned and ran off down the track. *So,* Denton thought.
He had seen the look in Cassidy's eye. *So there it is after all.*

Cassidy finished the rest of the ritual lap. Then it would be
off with the flats, on with the spikes, off with the damp T-shirt,
on with the nylon racing singlet: ritual ritual ritual. He had done
it exactly this way hundreds of times.

A roar came from the crowd that he did not understand.
Nothing was going on with the field events, and they were between races on the track. Then he looked over at the competitors' entrance and understood. A knot had formed, a chancre of
humanity around the gate that suddenly opened up and expelled
in a burst the fastest miler in history.

The crowd went crazy as he ambled easily across the track

with a wan smile, giving the stands a little wave. But Cassidy could tell, even from where he stood, the kind of look in his eye as he glanced quickly around the stadium and with a shudder dropped his bag to tug up the zipper on his turtleneck warm-up.

Little fluffs of hair on the back of Cassidy's neck went prickly again as Walton began his striders.

He was nearly two inches shorter than Cassidy but looked as if he could run through a wall. He already had his spikes on. Every eye in the place followed him as he began doing his sprints on the back straight. The black suit of New Zealand, Cassidy thought, the silver leaf—*Baillie, Halberg, Snell*. His idols, his gods! And now Walton.

Then he shook his head violently and swore under his breath at himself: *goddamn you!*

The roar had gone! He had been watching Walton slack-jawed like some high school kid and the roar in his own head had just gone! He jumped up, spikes on, and sprinted around the first turn, ignoring (not really seeing) Denton's bemused expression as he went by. When he slowed to a jog on the far side, calmer now, his jaw was set, his eyes fixed in a trance, and the orb rested inside a howling mindstorm. He did not realize that the figure flashing by on the turn had been Walton.

Now Cassidy took off his sweat bottoms, jogged around and left them at his bag; he kept the top on and jogged on. This was the way he always did it. They were getting ready to run off the high hurdles, the last race before the mile.

"THIRD CALL FOR THE MILE RUN. ALL MILERS REPORT TO THE STARTER."

The last leap of his heart jounced him as he heard the announcement but by now he was accustomed to the shock. He made no move for the starting line, nor did any of the other milers. The high hurdles hadn't even been run and there would be several minutes of confusion afterward while the timers sorted things out. The milers knew all these ancient rhythms, so they kept doing their striders and jogging. The gun cracked for the highs and they looked across the track at the race with the mildest sort of curiosity. After the hurdlers had swept past the finish line the announcer was after them again: "ALL MILERS REPORT TO THE STARTER IMMEDIATELY. LAST CALL FOR THE ONE-MILE RUN." It no longer jolted him because it was *all* jolt now. He barely heard the loudspeaker, such was the roar in his head. When he took off his sweat top he realized he had not put on his racing singlet. He was still in the wet T-shirt! *Goddamn it! How the hell could I have* . . .

Then he got control again, jogged rapidly over to his bag and changed. There was still plenty of time even though most of the milers were on the track milling around. The timers were in disarray from the previous race and the starter was walking among the runners as Cassidy knew he would. *"All right, gentlemen,"* he was saying, *"all right, listen to the starting instructions, gentlemen,"* as the runners paced back and forth, jiggling and jumping up and down, avoiding eyes, gasping their little shallow gasps, shaking out legs that didn't need shaking, and generally living their last few seconds of torment. Cassidy jogged out among them, feeling feathery light now in just racing nylon and spikes; he felt as though he weighed about ten pounds. He wore the white and blue Adidas 9.9s that had never been second.

Cassidy too took up the jiggling and pacing. The announcer was making introductions, but no one seemed to be paying attention. Walton was in lane one, so naturally they started with the outside lane. All eyes were on just one person, the powerful-looking Kiwi in the all-black nylon with a little silver fern over the breast. There was polite applause for the Finn in lane three, but when the announcer started on the final introduction, he didn't get to the gold medals, the world records, the endless titles, before the place was a madhouse. Everyone knew it all already. Walton jogged out a few steps and waved. Denton stood by the first turn in his navy blue USA team sweats, watching. *You have to learn the little smile and wave,* he thought, *that's one part of it maybe you don't think about beforehand. I'll bet that's the last thing old John wants to be doing right now. Even before a race like this.*

Cassidy thought, *Easy easy easy. Be careful through the turn and get through the first lap. Then start* thinking. *Easy easy easy. Save your goodies.*

"All right, gentlemen," the starter was saying in his executioner's tone, gun hanging down at the end of his fluorescent orange sleeve. "A two-command start, gentlemen, 'take your marks' and then the gun. Is that clear? All right, gentlemen, stand tall. Stand tall, gentlemen . . ."

The crowd hushed suddenly.

High up in the stands very nearly directly across from the starting post, Andrea sat beside the very excited umbrella man and thought, *It's him.*

The starter was backing out from among them now, still saying, "Stand tall, gentlemen, stand tall . . ."

And Quenton Cassidy stood tall in the night as a very slight breeze brushed his burning face. *At last,* he thought, *at last it is here. It is really here.*

The starter began backing off the track in quick little steps, raising his gun arm at the same time. For just an instant, Cassidy looked over to lane one and saw John Walton staring right back at him.

"TAKE YOUR MARKS!"

Cassidy's heart tried to leap out through his thin taut skin and hop into his wet hands. But outwardly it was all very calm, very serene, just as always, and it seemed to last a tiny forever, just like that, a snapshot of them all there on the curved parabola of a starting line, eight giant hearts attached to eight pairs of bellowslike lungs mounted on eight pairs of supercharged stilts. They were poised there on the edge of some howling vortex they had run ten thousand miles to get to. Now they had to run one more.

ℒ

CRACK!

There was the tiny little flutter during which he thought his legs were going to fail completely, but then they were away, out of their crouches and fairly bolting, bounding out and away, not even smoothly yet, burning off the first rush of excitement and fear. But here Cassidy found himself about two yards in front already and probably right on schedule for his maniac twenty-five-second 220. Standing on the inside of the curve, Denton flashed by and said quietly: tuck in. Cassidy tucked in.

He didn't recognize the green singlet, but it occurred to him that it had to be the runner in lane two. Walton was obviously behind them somewhere, unworried and unrushed. Then Cassidy glanced again and recognized the Irishman. Of course! He had hardly paid attention to anyone else in the race. The first 220 went by as always, giddily, and as they flashed by the white post someone gave them an unofficial split: 26.2 Yeeow! Too fast! No wonder Walton didn't hop right on up there. But there was no chance to look around; Cassidy could sense runners on his outside shoulder and twice he felt someone clipping his heel. He was running almost abreast of the Irishman, sharing the lead actually, but the real truth was that he was more surrounded than anything else. As they came out of the second turn he dared a quick glance to the inside and saw Walton, striding comfortably, head down, watching the feet flashing by in front of him; all business. Okay, thought Cassidy, stay right there. Right where you are.

It was an untenable attitude, he knew, but at this moment before it all got wild and bad it was easy to entertain such facile delusions of control. The crowd shrieked as they passed the starting post in a knot. But did he hear that? Probably not. He thought he heard one single shout: "Go Cassidy."

". . . fifty-SIX, fifty-SEVEN, fifty-EIGHT . . ." They were

going by the post. Denton, flashing by again on the inside, said quickly, "Fifty-seven five too fast." Remarkable, he said it almost in a conversational tone, but Cassidy heard it distinctly. All right, Bruce, it's too goddamn fast, what the hell am I supposed to do about it?

The announcer was saying: "O'RORK, THEN KAITAINEN, HARRIS, AND JOHN WALTON OF NEW ZEALAND . . ."

Then it started to come on him, as it always did here. He usually felt it in the gut first; a slow, acid kind of strain, systems beginning to panic down there; intestines, other organs closing down for the duration, preparing for whatever dire project was under way. And the legs now started to get the first wave of lactic acid numbness, the start of a deep ache that would all too soon become the ambulatory paralysis of the final straightaway. Even this early he was getting all the old feelings, thinking, *God, here it is again! Back in it again and I had forgotten completely what it was like. Forgotten altogether. Shoulders and arms starting now. Pay attention, goddamn it!*

The orb bobbed gently, taking it all in, retaining it, keeping it quiet inside the steely interior and allowing him to think. He concentrated on his task.

Even from the far straightaway he could hear the crowd grow uneasy and then erupt, but before he could react he sensed a body coming up on his shoulder and then flinging by to take the lead. A roar came from across the field. Cassidy pondered calmly, Who was it? It wasn't Walton. A short runner in all red. Wisconsin? St. Johns? He racked his brain, but came up with nothing. Was he a rabbit or just some guy looking for a few seconds of glory, leading John Walton in a mile? Cassidy hung where he was all through the turn coming into the home straight for the second time, then glanced back to the inside and saw Walton, this time a little more labored, but still running casually, eyes cast slightly downward, watching the feet in front of him. The roar was deafening as they went by, but this time he was sure he heard it, there was no mistake, several voices called out, "Go Cassidy!"

". . . one fifty-SEVEN, one fifty-EIGHT, one fifty-NINE . . ."

Then two things happened almost at once. First Bruce Denton flashed by, said calmly, *One fifty-seven good.* And a split second after that the crowd erupted again as a black-suited runner bolted by in a savage burst of speed: *WALTON! What the hell is he doing?* Cassidy thought.

The announcer, excited, came on: "AND NOW WALTON HAS TAKEN THE LEAD FROM HARRIS AS THEY WENT BY THE HALF IN . . ." Cassidy couldn't hear the rest.

Jesus, what is he doing? Cassidy thought as he watched the black-suited figure easily slide by the runner in red, and keep on, showing no sign of slowing down. Cassidy was really feeling it now, starting the third lap, the old intestine-sliding-down-the-leg extremis that comes at the precise middle of a race when it dawns on you that there is a long melancholy way to go. But there was Walton, *pulling away.*

Quenton Cassidy did not know it, of course, but here was the decision for all time, the decision that would lead him up the path to the higher callings or off on a side road to end up in the bushes somewhere. There was really no thinking to it; his face now set firmly in the race mask, showing nothing more than a detached strained interest, he let out a surge and found himself fairly flying around the Irishman down the back straight. Red shirt was already fading badly from his burst and Cassidy was by him quickly too. He pulled into lane one and thought, *That was too fast! You could have done that better.* But it was too late for recriminations. He set about hauling in the black suit in front of him, even now blending into the night, spikes flashing in a blur ahead. And this: from across the field, the calls, more of them, louder, most positive, beseeching now: "CASSIDY! CASSIDY!"

The announcer: ". . . WALTON OF NEW ZEALAND WITH KAITAINEN SEVEN YARDS BACK . . ."

His shoulders ached now with the heavy strain of lactic acid, so he pumped harder, concentrated on his form, trying to cover ground smoothly. Now was the time he wanted to be floating, covering ground with as little effort as possible, but he found himself straining just to hold pace. And Walton looked so easy! Was he of this earth? Could it really be this much of a joke to him, running this pace without a care in the world?

Cassidy could not feel his legs but that was all right. He was flying along in the night concentrating so hard on the black-suited demon out there that he was actually surprised to hit the second turn. He cursed mentally when he found himself flung by his own momentum out into the second lane, then got it under control, leaned into the turn and got back in rhythm. *A stupid mistake,* he thought, *and it cost me two yards.*

But coming out of the turn into the straight he felt it. He had contact. Walton had come back to him some and he had contact from five yards back. And he had the power. He knew that too as they sped down the straight, really feeling it now, the lactic acid aching through his body, but also starting the buildup, getting excited knowing that this time it would not be long, that it wasn't going to go on forever after all.

Down past the stands and this time Cassidy heard, unbelieving, what they were chanting as the two figures went by the white starting post: "CASS-A-DAY! CASS-A-DAY! CASS-A-DAY!"

Even the announcer no longer played the game: ". . . IT'S WALTON FOLLOWED BY . . . CASSIDY OF SOUTHEAST-ERN . . ."

Dick Doobey, nearly blind with rage, blood vessels standing out on his soft red face, jumped up from his seat in the officials' section and started out the gate onto the track to do God only knew what when he ran smack into the really quite startlingly muscled arm of Mike Mobley, that was stretched across the opening, his huge hand holding the far post in a death grip. Mobley challenged him for an instant with a gaze full of contempt and pity, then the giant turned back to the race and the chant: "CASS-A-DAY! CASS-A-DAY! CASS-A-DAY!"

His face ashen, Doobey slumped into the nearest seat he could find. Up in the press box, in icy silence, Steven C. Prigman turned to look at the gentlemen of the press, some of whom waited for his reaction; he smiled ruefully, turned back to the race.

And Denton flashing by now: two fifty-five flat. Wait.

Then the gun: CRACK! And the hair on the back of his neck standing up as it always did. Cassidy thought, *Four hundred yards to go Jesus God what a cost just to be here and he's slipping away if I could just hold him now he's been flat out for . . .*

But Walton was not flat out at all. He suddenly looked back at Cassidy and Cassidy thought he saw a tiny flicker in those hard eyes: surprise. Not concern. Just a mild kind of surprise.

And that followed by a little burst so powerful and quick it broke Cassidy's heart. *God, how can he do that?*

Quenton Cassidy, sadly now, was starting to tie up halfway down the back straight and all he could think was: *Son of a bitch, what has he been doing running from the front? He never does that.* Now Cassidy's arms and shoulders were getting worse and worse as the orb strained and bounced around inside, trying to hold it all, Cassidy feeling now the process of his form starting to degenerate involuntarily, wanly remarked to himself that this must be how death is, *and look how easy dear God he looks up there. So this is how it is, this is exactly how it is, how he beats you and beats you and beats you.*

She had stood by with everyone else the last time, and though she knew umbrella man was unobtrusively observing her reactions now, she studied Cassidy's face when he went by and saw in it the totally dispassionate look of the runner at his toil; alert but not excited, full of strain and some unnamed misery, but so obviously showing no emotion, masking darker secrets. What was it he had said about demons? She had some idea of what Cassidy and Walton were experiencing because the other runners, some twenty yards behind, did not hold it as well as these two. Walton to her looked simply intimidating, as if he had been born at full stride; his torso was powerful for a runner and his every stride suggested merciless strength held in reserve. He was haughty in his power and it was somehow chilling to watch.

But then she had looked at Quenton Cassidy, saw the same objective, emotionless look about him, watched the sleek, machinelike workings of legs that were longer than Walton's. And suddenly she had seen him from a different perspective: he too looked intimidating. And something very deep inside her stirred as she realized that she was, after all, frightened for him, for this task he had taken upon himself. Her eyes had flooded and she stood there in her confusion and turmoil, not caring that umbrella man was staring at her.

"CASS-A-DAY! CASS-A-DAY! CASS-A-DAY!"

He was starting to get the white haze even this early; it would be very bad when it all caught up, but of course that was no consideration now. *Come on, you son of a bitch,* he thought, but he knew he was just hanging on. It was all going slowly downhill and Walton had about eight yards on him still. Cassidy could feel the muscles in his neck start to tighten, pulling his lower lip downward into an ugly grimace; he knew this was one of the last signs, this death sneer. *So this is what happens! You just don't get him, that's all! The son of a bitch just keeps on going and it ends and you don't get him ever!*

Cassidy adjusted his lean a little forward; that seemed to help some, but the neck was getting tighter and he felt his arms beginning to stiffen. By the time they got out of the turn and into the last straight, he knew they would be really bad. All down the back straight Cassidy tried to reel him in, but it was no good. Eight yards. Eight yards, *eight yards*! The strain was apparent to those close to the track; on the exhale breath he made little gasps: *gahh! gahh! gahh!* His eyes were starting to squeeze up shut but he could hardly see through the white haze anyway.

The chant roared across the field, beseeching, hopeful, frenzied.

"CASS-A-DAY! CASS-A-DAY! CASS-A-DAY!"

Shut up! Shut up! I'm not your goddamn hero! All down the back straight he stared at the fleeing black suit through the wrinkled slits his eyes had become, stared at the black suit and wished they would all leave him alone. Just leave him the hell alone with his misery and defeat.

That's when he saw it.

Almost imperceptible, but there it was just the same: the left shoulder dipped suddenly, then the right leg shot out a little farther than usual, and that was it: back to normal stride.

Walton was tying up too.

So that's the way it is. Not so casual after all.

Cassidy bore down, bore down, and finally began reeling him in, all during the final turn, all the way around he pulled him in, inch by inch, as his mouth was drawn more and more into the ugly grimace by the spastic neck muscles. Inch by inch the black suit came back until finally they broke clear of the turn and there it was: John Walton was three feet ahead of him with a hundred and ten yards of Tartan stretching out in front of them to the finish line. There was utter pandemonium in the stands as the chant degenerated into a howling, shrieking din.

Quenton Cassidy moved out to the second lane, the Lane of High Hopes, and ran out the rest of the life in him.

37

A Stiller Town

ALL THROUGH THE LAST FIFTY YARDS he had looked through the two fogged slits of windows at the howling slow-motion nightmare going on around him as his body rigged up in true fashion, getting the jaw-shoulder lock and the sideways final straight fade and he began to lose all semblance of control. He peered out at all this as the orb was about to burst, letting all the poison flood out, peered at it and quite calmly wondered, *When will it all end?*

He felt more than saw Walton come back up to his shoulder, entertained an idle curiosity about who would get it, but then went back to wistfully concentrating on those green inches of Tartan passing slowly, slowly beneath his feet.

The last ten yards his body was a solid block of lactic acid, with those straining neck muscles pulling his lip down and his back arched, trapezia trying to pull him over backward. And all the way Quenton Cassidy was telling himself:

Not now . . . it hurts but go all the way through do not stop until you are past it you cannot afford to give the son of a bitch anything . . . so holdit holdit holdit Jesus Christ hold it holditholditHOLDITHOLDIT-HOLD IT . . .

Finally with a scream and a violent wrenching motion he shook himself loose from this terrible force that gripped him, made himself bend into a semblance of a lean and it was over . . .

. . . OR AT LEAST HE THOUGHT it was over if it was not all some bad dream and he is gasping simply wrenching air from around him feeling death surely imminent here beside him crying and going hands to knees, stumbling please leave me, please I don't want, please I need to breathe . . .

And then Denton has him around the waist and is lifting him up off the ground, please Bruce put me down I can't breathe but Denton is taking him off, away from them, dragging the tall brown limp doll which apparently cannot stand on its own, holding him up painfully and saying, Remember it, Quenton, goddamn you better remember it because it doesn't ever get any better, are you listening to me, goddamn you? and Cassidy forcing his eyes open finally and seeing Denton through the white haze and seeing that he is crying too. Oh Bruce I'm listening please let me go Jesus it hurts and Denton lets him go hands to knees to pray to the runner's finish line god but Denton leans over and whispers: three fifty-two five, Cass. He kicked from five hundred yards out but it was you, Quenton Cassidy, it was YOU all the way. You know you beat him, don't you, Quenton, goddamn it?

But Cassidy can't do anything but hold his knees and make his little gagging noises and nod, wishing everyone would just leave him the hell alone so he could see if he was going to die.

WALTON WALKS BY and they touch hands; Walton regards Cassidy with curiosity but no fear. He nods to Denton.

"Bruce," he says.

"John."

This is no game for upstarts or big surprises and Walton's look is clearly more of curiosity than anything else. There will be time, his eyes say, time for decisions and revisions.

"Later, mate," he says to Quenton Cassidy. A respectful nod to Denton and he is gone.

Later, Cassidy says to himself.

When, after the countless flashes of cameras and the rude pushing, the well-wishing, and the endless questions (still wanting to know *The Secret*), after all of that he finally got away from them and talked with Bruce Denton quietly for a few moments; he pulled the zipper up all the way on the sweat top against the evening chill and stepped out onto the track as those remaining in the bleachers roared. Quenton Cassidy looked up, gave a little smile and wave and thought, *I have nowhere to go.*

It was then that Bruce Denton turned with a sigh and walked alone toward the gate, thinking that Quenton Cassidy's smile looked sad indeed . . .

38.

. . . A Runner

THE YOUNG MAN WALKED STEADILY through the far turn, the darkest part of the track, and entered the final straightaway. Here, he thought, it is usually all over; just a matter of throwing what is left into it. It would be exciting to the onlookers perhaps, but the runners would be calmly playing it out.

During the second and third laps he had tried to conjure up the old feeling of despair and pain, but as always could not quite get it. It had to be experienced, not remembered.

Now he was walking the last fifty yards, unconsciously swinging his arms a little more vigorously, trying to conjure up some of that helpless frozen broth of the last few yards, when the arms and shoulders, legs and hips, all seem to bind themselves up together and the jaw locks into the tight grimace as if in supplication, and all of life is reduced to a simple desperation, a pleading for the last pathetic twitch from simple clay. How well he knew these things.

Then he was by the post, telling himself for the last five yards, Go *through it,* go all the way through it. He stopped and looked around. The pain would catch you here, of course, the orb would shatter as soon as you crossed the line and it would overwhelm you for those first few seconds. That, of all the feelings, was the one that your mind protected you from the most; later you wouldn't even be able to get a hint of it.

But he supposed that even as bad as it was then, there must be some kind of pleasure mixed in with it, some desperate relief. Joy, perhaps, in knowing that it was over, one more time, with nothing held back.

He took several deep breaths of the warm September air and then walked to the infield to get his travel bag. He looked around once more at the vaulting pits, the oblong sandbox of the horizontal jumpers, the concrete rings for the weight men, and finally back at the starting post. His eyes then took in the track, slowly following the rubberized surface all the way around the first turn, down the long lonely back straight past the 220 post, around the far turn, and then back up the final straight to the finish post where he had long ago beaten the great John Walton. Uncomplicated dimensions that had for some years now defined his life.

A quarter of a mile that he knew by the inches. There was much to be left behind here, he thought. But I can live with that.

He walked straight across the infield, across the track, and out the gate, leaving the joggers to their nightly toil. The moths still worried the streetlight.

The young man stopped momentarily amid the dancing insect shadows and opened the small travel bag. He reached around under the passport, clothes, and toilet articles until he found it. He opened the flat, thin oblong box under the streetlight and looked at it once more.

The heavy round disk reposed against pink satin, its thick purple ribbon curling up and behind the soft material. The writing around the edge was in Greek but the general import was clear enough.

In the pale light the silver metal glowed dully. It no longer stabbed at him.

This I can live with too, he thought. Primarily because I no longer have any say in the matter. He smiled faintly, closed the box, and replaced it in the bottom of the bag. He turned without looking back and walked away from the track.

There was a very old gnarled tree somewhere he wanted to find and then he would be on his way.

Afterword

More than thirty years have passed since Quenton Cassidy and his teammates first took to the streets of the fictional Kernsville to get in their miles for the day. Go back a few more years and you would find the actual runners who inspired their literary counterparts, striding the very real sidewalks and trails of Gainesville, Florida, and the 440-yard track at the University of Florida.

It would be a base cliché to say that the world has remade itself since then, and it's not altogether true anyway. Modern athletes aren't being harassed or excommunicated for sporting long hair or shirts without collars (as they most certainly were then), but young Americans are still dying in far-off lands for ill-defined and dubious reasons, and millions of citizens of the Republic still believe that whoever did or did not prevail on the gridiron last Saturday is of the utmost consequence to mankind.

On the other hand, women athletes—all but nonexistent in Quenton's day—delightfully now abound, runners are commonplace on America's sidewalks, and consider this: On the afternoon of September 30, 1968, your faithful scribe ran in a cross-country race with a friend and teammate from West Palm Beach named Johnnie Brown, who thus became the first black athlete in history to compete for the University of Florida.

So the world is indeed a different place than it was in Quenton's time, yet the verities he pursued and the standards by which he lived remain unsullied by time's withering touch.

That we can even contemplate these things now is due to the simple fact that all those years ago I yearned to read a book like *Once a Runner* and found that it did not exist. It was a strange sensation, longing for a book that no one had yet written, but it slowly dawned on me that I might be able to do something about that. I came to believe that it might be possible to capture some of the bittersweet beauty and heartbreak of the only all-consuming quest for physical excellence I would likely experience in my lifetime.

When I had finished writing the book and felt that it just might be worthwhile, I found that many, many people involved in the publishing and selling of books felt altogether otherwise. And thus the volume you hold in your hands came perilously close to never existing at all.

But distance runners are nothing if not determined and the book was in fact born all those years ago. It endures today and Kernsville remains alive in the minds and imaginations of many generations of runners and readers.

And though time may indeed have slowed or even stilled the light-foot lads upon whom the characters were based, it is a great comfort to me to know that Quenton Cassidy is still somewhere out there on the ethereal trails with Denton and Mizner, Benny Vaughn, Nubbins, and the rest, laughing at somebody's silly joke, imagining great victories, teasing the new guy.

But putting in their miles, always.

John L. Parker, Jr.
October 2009
Bar Harbor, Maine

A SCRIBNER

READING GROUP GUIDE

Once a Runner
John L. Parker, Jr.

Introduction

A classic novel and a particular favorite among runners and track teams, *Once a Runner* is the story of Quenton Cassidy, a collegiate runner who specializes in the mile. When Quenton becomes involved with a petition protesting the athletic department's dress and conduct code, he is suspended from the track team and prohibited from competing in the university's annual track meet.

Following the advice of his Olympian mentor, Bruce Denton, Quenton gives up his scholarship, his girlfriend, and perhaps his future by taking to a monastic retreat in the countryside to train. The seclusion and regimen bring Quenton to the very brink of his physical and mental limits, but it all seems worth it when Denton suggests a plan that could allow him to compete against the best miler in the world. As a man who actually lived and trained with gold medalists and world record holders, John L. Parker, Jr., presents a rare insider's glimpse at the incredibly intense lives of elite distance runners.

Questions and Topics for Discussion

1. "Time reposed in peculiar receptacles; to him the passing of one minute took on all manner of rare meaning" (p. 2). Dis-

cuss the theme of subjective time that pervades the novel. How does Quenton manipulate his own conceptions of time in order to master the psychological aspects of training and competing?

2. The colorful character Sidecar Doobey has little to do with sports or running. What does he add to the story?

3. There are many animal metaphors scattered throughout the novel, along with the idea of running as a primal human activity. Does Cassidy recognize these aspects of his sport, and if so, what is his attitude toward them?

4. The narrator suggests that Jerry Mizner's obsessive-compulsive personality meant that "his mind adapted well to the distance runner's daily toil" while Quenton's spontaneity meant that he must "painfully teach himself the . . . mentality of a dedicated runner" (p. 29). How does the discussion of nature versus nurture evolve in this context? Do you think Jerry would have needed the focused environment of a retreat as much as Quenton apparently did in order to succeed?

5. Quenton is clearly an intelligent student devoted to rationality and reason, yet he is hard put to explain his passion for running. Why do you suppose that is?

6. How do the playful dynamics of the team atmosphere affect the runners? What does Quenton lose when he leaves it behind? What does he gain?

7. Andrea's relationship with Quenton provides an example of an outsider to the running world sincerely trying to understand it. "And suddenly she had seen him from a different perspective: he too looked intimidating. And something very deep inside her stirred as she realized that she was, after all, frightened for him, for this task he had taken upon himself" (p. 265). What has Andrea suddenly understood from this new perspective? Why does it frighten her?

8. What is the significance of Quenton's childhood encounter

with death? During his recovery he tells his father he saw a bull shark in the water: "When he saw me he acted like he didn't care but he moved over a little to let me pass by. I was so ferocious with my sling, Dad, I wasn't afraid. I laughed because he was going so far in and I knew the hunting was better out near the tip" (p. 190). Why did this incident make Quenton feel powerful, and how does that feeling inform his running?

9. Bruce Denton plays a huge role in Quenton's progress as a runner. It is clear that he uses his own experiences to help Quenton train mentally and physically. In the end, he sees his own sad smile reflected on Quenton's face. Do you think Quenton and Bruce will share the same emotional fate? Why or why not?

10. Coach Doobey and President Prigman become stubborn obstacles for Quenton. Despite their best efforts, Quenton still manages to achieve his objective. What might a reader learn from how he goes about accomplishing his goals?

11. During Bruce's masochistic interval workout, he says, "This is where you find out. This is the time and place. All the rest is window dressing" (p. 222). When Quenton has finished, he says, "It is a very hard thing to have to know" (p. 226). What has he found out? Why is it so difficult to know?

12. When Quenton remembers Allan, the little boy he encountered while racing, he wonders "what it was about that one" (p. 253), the same thought his own father had about him. What about this child do you think touched Quenton so deeply? How does the fact that the boy was clearly disabled and yet was still able to partially mirror Quenton play into the novel?

13. The final race of this novel provides an extreme climax to Quenton's training. Why do you think it took a sign of Walton's vulnerability for Quenton to muster the strength to

catch him (p. 266)? How does that relate to the bull shark story mentioned earlier? What motivated him in those last fifty yards?

14. When Quenton returns as a silver medalist, he goes back to the track and finally indicates that "there was a very old gnarled tree somewhere he wanted to find" (p. 272). Earlier in the novel, Quenton mentions the tree while waiting for Andrea and thinks, "What does this old fellow care about it all? The strength of the ancient tree somehow soothed his misery" (p. 195). What does this tree represent for Quenton? What does it say about his attitude toward a future without running, a future not so bound up in distances and times?

Tips to Enhance Your Book Club

1. *Runner's World* offers an open forum for readers of *Once a Runner*. Read others' thoughts and add your own!
   http://opensource.runnersworld.com/2009/01/how-has-once-a.html

2. Start or join a runners' group in your area.
   http://www.coolrunning.com

3. Enter a race! Look up races of all lengths across the country.
   http://www.runnersworld.com/cda/racefinder

4. Learn more about the USA Olympic runners.
   http://www.teamusa.org

Read on for an excerpt from

Again to Carthage

Coming soon in paperback from Scribner

1

Newberry Redux

The cabin sat back off the road in the dripping trees like a part of the forest itself, earthy brown and plain, with a skin of cedar shakes, organic but for its giveaway straight edges. In the gloomy afternoon downpour the familiar shape seemed the essence of refuge.

Could it possibly have been just a year? Yes, and some days.

The screened-in front porch wasn't latched and he had already retrieved the front door key from his shaving kit where it had been for more than a year. Cassidy backed in dragging two big canvas equipment bags, disturbing spiders at work, breathing in the familiar scents of raw lumber, mildew, and the pepper and loamy decay of Spanish moss and north Florida piney forest. The place was perpetually unfinished inside, with stacks of building materials lying around and wiring showing in bare stud walls. Bruce wasn't kidding; he hadn't been out in a long time.

He dropped his gear in the chaos of the so-called living room and just stood there with his eyes closed, the cascading scents of an earlier life making him dizzy with nostalgia.

As the rain deflected slightly off the steep sides of the A-frame, it seemed to him that this was the kind of day that seemed to happen in your life when Something Big had just ended. He flashed on a day from his central Florida childhood, the last day of the school year in junior high; he was waiting for a ride in the tropical downpour under the bus shelter in the empty parking lot. Everyone was gone and he could feel his aloneness settling over him like a damp shroud. There were parties going on somewhere, he thought. Ordinarily, a summer stretching out in front of him like a small infinity of freedom would have filled him with primal kid joy, but he was just plain morose.

His father was late, but it wasn't unusual in the days of one-car families for kids to spend a lot of time waiting for grown-ups. His occasional bouts of melancholia made no sense to him. He put his stupid decal-covered three-ring binder on the ground and lay on his back on the concrete bench, contemplating a wasp's nest buzzing electronically overhead. He had not made any teams and he wasn't one of the cool kids and most of the teachers couldn't remember his name. That didn't bother him but what *really* got to him was the sudden revelation that this rainy nothing day was what all of life eventually came to, that everything sooner or later devolved to a point somewhere on the gray horizon where you're just some sad kid waiting alone in the rain.

Now, standing alone again in the cabin as a young man, he had experienced a number of such rainy End-of-Something days in his life. But because he was still young and little touched by death these days often had to do with school years or athletic seasons.

Back before it all happened, during all those long days, nights, weeks, months, and years of training, he thought of the future as a kind of foggy diorama. If everything turned out the way it was supposed to, his later life would be some kind of stroll with a desirable female into the middle distance, a happy American epilogue befitting the narrative line, inspiring music crescendoing into the Warner Bros. logo, a glad coda for a three-act culture.

But he had always kept it nebulous in his head, and now that the time had come he found that the girl had actually married someone else and gone away and he had not Won the Big Race and he would not grace any cereal boxes. Also, he didn't know how to stroll and there was no music except for one eerily chipper Gilbert O'Sullivan ditty he could not turn off in his head, something about climbing a tower and launching yourself into the indifferent void. Standing there in the familiar musty half-light of a late-summer thunderstorm, he thought, It's just like the lady always said: No bugles, no drums.

The small television set was where he had left it in the oven, cord wrapped round and round. A bunch of books were still stacked next to the cot in the small bedroom in the back: *A Fan's Notes, The Bushwhacked Piano, Zen and the Art*. He had done a lot of reading out here as he lolled around between workouts, trying to coax his body back to life so he could go out and carefully brutalize it again.

Loll. That was the word for it. Time lolled away napping, thinking, daydreaming, waiting for his damaged corpuscles to rearrange themselves into a more perfect union.

He went to the plate-glass window at the front of the cabin and, sure enough, down in one corner were the faint dusty outlines of the words he had written in reversed mirror script on the foggy pane one lonely winter afternoon long ago: *Help. Imprisoned in February*.

I should unpack, he thought. I should make the bed, get this place organized, *something*. But there it was: no ambition. At all at all.

So, he did what he had done so many thousands of times before when his life was at loose ends and he didn't have a thought in his head: He pulled on his togs and blew out the front door and was hitting right at six-minute pace before the screen door had even finished double-slamming behind him.

His battered lemon-yellow 914 was still clicking in the cool rain as he splashed down the rutty red-clay drive that always reminded him of North Carolina. He turned at the blacktop and after a quick half mile veered off at the familiar trailhead and disappeared into the forest. He had felt so logy that he was surprised his legs loosened up quickly on the carpet of pine needles, and it wasn't long before he fell into a miler's tempo stride and began clipping miles off at not much slower than five-minute pace. It was much too fast for overdistance, he knew, but he wasn't training anymore. He was just running.

The trail went deep into the endless stand of blackjack pine and water oak and up by Otter Springs and then almost all the way down upon the Suwannee River, where in fact very few old folks stay. Four miles into the run at the bottom of a gentle rise he called Blackberry Hill he was startled to see his own ghostly footprints at the edge of the trail. He remembered the day he had made them long ago. It was rainy like this and he was skirting a big puddle, trying to keep his shoes dry as long as he could. Strange to think the evidence of his ephemeral passing would still be here hardened into the earth, partially hidden by encroaching weeds, like poor little Lucy's footprints on that plain in Africa, still there after three million years. Taking the hill with big strides he thought: We never really know what will happen to the scratches we make in this thin dust.

Familiarity made the trail go by quickly and he blinked back from a daydream having to do with billfishing in the Gulf Stream to realize he was almost finished. Good thing too, with the glistening woods now darkening before his eyes. Eight miles and he hadn't seen a living soul. He had seen a herd of deer, a probable wild turkey—at the distance he couldn't be sure—a red-tailed hawk, and several mullet evading predators or just jumping for joy.

He finished, as usual, going hard down the last perfectly straight row of Sidecar Doobey's pecan grove, the flat grass inviting speed and bringing on the old fantasy of being in the final straight of the Olympic 1500, straining to reach the leader, leaning for the tape and reminding oneself over and over: go *through* the tape, go all the way through it, with nothing held back. Just like the old days when he would be out there with Mizner and the guys, running along the sidewalks of Kernsville in pretend slow motion as the half-miler Benny Vaughn did his mock-serious announcer, giving them all funny foreignized names to make them sound more glamorous, doing the play-by-play as they made agonistic faces and leaned histrionically toward the imaginary finish line. Benny had named him Quintus Cassadamius, the famous Greek miler. It struck him for the first time just now—and with a quick flare of pride—that a new generation of dreamy kids might now accord him his own name. In these mock race scenarios Bruce Denton had no glitzed-up fantasy name, a gold medal being about as glamorous as you could get in their little world. Cassidy wondered now if maybe a near miss was worth something too.

Funny, he thought, I was there in real life yet running down this lane I go back to the same old fantasy. We few who get to experience both eventually find out that the real thing and the fantasy can coexist in your head. He would love to tell the undergraduates about that. It was the kind of thing they would talk about for hours on training runs. Mize, Nubbins, Burr, Atkinson, Schiller. Old dour Hosford. They were mostly gone now, graduated or otherwise scattered. Off to wars, other schools, wives. Where oh where, he wondered, are my light-foot lads? What has become of *the old team*?

He jogged in from the highway using the long driveway as a cool down and was glad he had left the porch light on, dark as it was getting. He toed off the muddy shoes and left them outside, fetching a dry towel from the bedroom but returning to the porch to continue dripping. It wouldn't do any good to shower yet, he would just start sweating again, so he plopped down in an aluminum lawn chair and watched the rainy night come on. He had been wet so long his fingertips were wrinkled. Steam rose from his skin.

He didn't know if it was bad yet. Bruce said it would get very bad before it got better. That was just part of it. The big buildup and then the *really* big letdown. Worse than you could ever imagine.

Truth be told, though, at this moment he was feeling pretty darn good.

He was through with the Trial of Miles, the quest that had consumed him these past umpteen years. He was wet and hungry and, in a general epistemological sense, adrift. He was sitting on a borrowed porch at the end of the road at the end of the summer at the end of his athletic career, dripping salty rainwater in a perimeter around a cheap aluminum chair. And he was once again staring into the moist gloom of Marjorie's ancient piney flatwoods.

But twenty-seven miles away back in Kernsville catty corner from the campus was a white-columned faux southern mansion that housed the University City Bank, an establishment founded by Sidecar Doobey's old man with the obscene profits he made running rum on shrimp boats from Key West up the west coast of Florida to Apalachicola, thence to Tallahassee and Atlanta on the seafood trains, bonded booze disguised by a scant layer of ice and red snapper, but in actuality protected by a well-paid bridge of crooks stretching from Monroe County all the way to Washington, D.C.

That bank had been his last stop before heading out to Newberry that afternoon. It contained a safe-deposit box, number 1347, newly opened in the name of Quenton Cassidy and paid for a year in advance, the key now dangling from the fresh-air lever of the beat-up Porsche in the front yard. Box 1347 was in the lower left-hand corner of the far wall of the vault. It was the smallest size offered. The slide-out metal drawer held only one item: a flat oblong leather box.

In that box was an Olympic silver medal.

2

Breakfast Game

F ried green tomatoes . . ."

"Good one."

". . . with freshly ground red, black, and white pepper in the batter!"

"Very good one. Some of these southern delicacies have grown on me and that's one of them. How about this one: generous hunks of freshly cut pineapple . . ."

"Oooooh . . ." Cassidy's saliva glands jumped.

". . . served on a bed of shaved ice!"

The midmorning sun was baking the steam out of the glistening landscape, but not unpleasantly so, as they made their way along the trail at an easy pace, playing the Breakfast Game, which meant they would soon be driving around looking for a Shoney's.

"Okay, here's one and this will probably do it for me: cheese grits . . ."

"*No grits!*"

"Yes, cheese grits, real ones not instant, with salt and pepper and a little melted butter on top, but here's the kicker: Interspersed throughout are chunks of that thick brown-sugar-cured bacon."

"Hmmm. Bacon you say?"

"Brown-sugar-cured and cooked not too long, just nice and firm."

Denton considered this.

"Okay, as long as you put in the bacon. The grits then become just a transport medium for the cured meat and the dairy product."

Such is the guiltless chitchat of rare-as-iridium beings with less than 5 percent body fat. They ran along in comfortable silence, lost in thoughts of buttery dishes. When they reached the bottom of Blackberry Hill the undergrowth closed in on the trail so that even going single-file they both got a good chilly brushing with wet leaves from both sides.

"Ick. Trail's not gotten a lot of use lately," said Denton.

"Guess not," Cassidy agreed. "You look like you're in shape, but obviously not from running out here."

"Nope. Been sticking close to home working on the ol' thesis. Getting in some miles, though. The heels have been better lately. I've been thinking about racing a little."

They ran along in silence for a while. Then Denton asked, "Cass, are you really sure you want to be out here?"

"What do you mean?"

"Staying out here at the A-frame, away from everything."

"Why not?"

"It's just maybe not such a good time to be alone."

Cassidy considered this. Denton had never told Cassidy a single important thing that had not sooner or later turned out to be true.

"There has been something of a letdown," Cassidy admitted. "I know you warned me, but I honestly didn't think it would be this bad. It's a weird feeling . . ."

"I know."

"Kind of empty, you know?"

"Yep. It can get pretty bad."

"I've had a few bad days, but I'm all right. I've survived blue funk before."

"Well, I've talked to a lot of guys and it's pretty typical no matter how you did, win lose or draw. The thing itself is so cathartic, so *final,* that hardly anyone in the Games will have thought much beyond it. I read that somewhere, but I didn't understand it until I went through it. Come to think of it, it's one of the reasons that every one of you is there on the starting line in the first place. It's the single-mindedness that got you there."

"We definitely know our way around deferred gratification," Cassidy said.

"It's your *life* you've been deferring, Cass. That comes crashing in on you. Maybe it hasn't really hit you yet, but it will. You're maybe still sort of in the slipstream of it all, the hoopla, the interviews, the boondoggle invitations, flying around, your relatives calling to say they saw you on TV . . ."

"I think I'm out of the slipstream already," said Cassidy glumly. "Maybe that's the hidden blessing of coming second. Anyway, that's one of the reasons I wanted to come back here. I wanted something familiar."

"Ah, yes. It helps to have something to come back to, that's for sure," said Denton. "Well, you're welcome out here. You know that."

Another silent mile went by.

"Heard anything from Mize?" Denton said.

"He's doing flight training in Texas. Helicopters. Says he

loves it. I sure hope the whole mess is over before he goes over there and does something stupid."

"I don't know if it's ever going to be over. What happened to the Army track thing?"

"He decided against it. Thought it would be copping out. He doesn't think much of the war, but he's strange about these things. You know what he also considered?"

"What?"

"Being a medic."

Denton whistled.

"He's always been like that. He wasn't in ROTC to line up a deferment either. In his own weird way, Mize has always been a kind of true believer. In another age he would have been a Quaker or something. But no. No track dodge for him. I'm sure they offered it to him."

"And no medic. Helicopters."

"Helicopters. Little ones. With guns on them."

"Well, to change the subject only slightly, what did you decide about school?"

"I'm going to go. I can't think of anything better to do. There's no deferment, of course, and I don't have a family like you so I have no idea what I'm going to do about that, but I haven't been called up for my physical yet, so I'm going to at least start it."

"Where?"

"I'm thinking of staying here. At first it was just my backup, but I think I've changed my mind. Duke and Vandy are better law schools, but right now I can't imagine picking up and going to some new place. I'm thinking of taking some time off and starting winter quarter. They're being incredibly nice to me at Tigert Hall for some reason. I'm apparently no longer considered just a pain-in-the-ass loudmouth from a nonrevenue sport."

"Public opinion's shifting. Even Cronkite has turned. McNamara'll go to his grave saying our so-called police action was the only way to stop global blah blah. But he'll be the only one. But hey!"

"Yeah?"

"Want some advice?"

"No."

"Go ahead and start school now. Take some time later if you need to, but start now."

"Okay."

"I'm serious."

"I know."

"It will make it easier."

"Okay."

"And remember what Jumbo Elliot used to tell the Villanova guys."

"What was that?"

"Live like a clock."

"Live like a clock."

"Right."

"Live like a clock."

"That's what I said."

"Okay, I give up. I find Jumbo opaque at best. Where did you get this anyway?"

"Liquori. What Jumbo meant was keep to your schedule. If your morning run was always at eight A.M., you go out and do a token run at eight A.M., even if you're tapering for a big race or on summer break. You're not really training, you're just keeping your body on the same routine. Eat at the same time, sleep at the same time. Live like a clock."

"Like Mussolini's widow."

"How's that?"

"After the war she'd go work in the fields from sunup to sundown. People would say, Why do you do that? She'd say, It's good hard work and when you do it all day you can sleep at night."

"I guess."

"So this is like I've just seen my spouse strung up upside down with his mistress by an angry mob after losing a world war? That what you're saying?"

"No, I'm saying live like a clock."

Cassidy gave him a sideways look.

"Think about this," Denton said. "A man with a hundred-dollar bill and a day to live might conceivably—under the right circumstances—have himself a wonderful time."

"Okay," Cassidy said, dubiously.

"But a man with a hundred-dollar bill and a week to live might well be in serious trouble."

"Anyone with a week to live is undoubtedly in serious trouble, regardless of his finances," Cassidy said.

"Context, Cass," said Denton. "Context and chronology are everything. Timing, if you will."

"I don't like it when you start 'if you willing,'" Cassidy said glumly.

"You've capitalized yourself mightily to this point," Denton said. "For years and years now, putting everything in, taking nothing out." He gestured at the trail in front of them, as if it represented all their trials and all their miles.

"But it's perfectly okay to live your life a little now, Quenton," he continued. "You've earned *at least* that much. No one will blame you, no one will fault you. Everything doesn't have to hurt, everything doesn't have to be a battle."

Cassidy snorted. "How would *you* possibly know—"

"I *know!*" Denton said, too loudly. They ran in silence for a while, Cassidy thinking to himself, Oh Jesus, what an addlepate I can be.

"I wish someone had been there to tell me," Denton said, quietly.

"Mmmm?"

"To live like a clock."

"Okay, Bruce."

They ran quietly again. Finally, Cassidy said: "Bruce, I've been doing that very thing for *years* now . . ."

"Exactly!"

"I've lived like a clock for nearly four years in college, through quitting school and racing Walton, through the buildup for the trials, and then right to the finals of the goddamn Olympic 1500 meters."

"Right."

"And you're telling me . . ."

"To keep doing it."